Gastroenterology

Editor

PARVATHI PERUMAREDDI

PRIMARY CARE: CLINICS IN OFFICE PRACTICE

www.primarycare.theclinics.com

Consulting Editor
JOEL J. HEIDELBAUGH

September 2023 • Volume 50 • Number 3

ELSEVIER

1600 John F. Kennedy Boulevard • Suite 1800 • Philadelphia, Pennsylvania, 19103-2899

http://www.theclinics.com

PRIMARY CARE: CLINICS IN OFFICE PRACTICE Volume 50, Number 3
September 2023 ISSN 0095-4543, ISBN-13: 978-0-443-18368-3

Editor: Taylor Hayes
Developmental Editor: Jessica Cañaberal

Primary Care: Clinics in Office Practice (ISSN: 0095-4543) is published quarterly by Elsevier Inc., 360 Park Avenue South, New York, NY 10010-1710. Months of issue are March, June, September, and December. Periodicals postage paid at New York, NY and additional mailing offices. Subscription prices are $277.00 per year (US individuals), $629.00 (US institutions), $100.00 (US students), $321.00 (Canadian individuals), $712.00 (Canadian institutions), $100.00 (Canadian students), $379.00 (international individuals), $712.00 (international institutions), and $175.00 (international students). Foreign air speed delivery is included in all *Clinics* subscription prices. All prices are subject to change without notice. POSTMASTER: Send address changes to *Primary Care: Clinics in Office Practice*, Elsevier Periodicals Customer Service, 11830 Westline Industrial Drive, St. Louis, MO 63146. Customer Service Health Sciences Division, Subscription Customer Service, 3251 Riverport Lane, Maryland Heights, MO 63043. **Customer Service: 1-800-654-2452 (U.S. and Canada); 314-447-8871 (outside U.S. and Canada). Fax: 314-447-8029. E-mail: journalscustomerservice-usa@elsevier.com (for print support); journalsonlinesupport-usa@elsevier.com (for online support).**

Reprints. For copies of 100 or more, of articles in this publication, please contact the Commercial Reprints Department, Elsevier Inc., 360 Park Avenue South, New York, NY 10010-1710. Tel. 212-633-3874; Fax: 212-633-3820; E-mail: reprints@elsevier.com.

Primary Care: Clinics in Office Practice is covered in *MEDLINE/PubMed (Index Medicus) and EMBASE/ Excerpta Medica, Current Contents/Clinical Medicine, and ISI/BIOMED.*

Contributors

CONSULTING EDITOR

JOEL J. HEIDELBAUGH, MD, FAAFP, FACG
Clinical Professor, Departments of Family Medicine and Urology, Director of Medical Student Education and Clerkship Director, Department of Family Medicine, University of Michigan Medical School, Ann Arbor, Michigan; Ypsilanti Health Center, Ypsilanti, Michigan

EDITOR

PARVATHI PERUMAREDDI, DO
Associate Professor, Department of Medicine, Florida Atlantic University, Charles E. Schmidt College of Medicine-Florida Atlantic University, Boca Raton, Florida

AUTHORS

DALAL ALHAQQAN, MBBCh
Clinical Fellow, Division of Gastroenterology and Hepatology, MedStar Georgetown University Hospital, Washington, DC

MIRTHA Y. AGUILAR-ALVARDO, MD, MPH
Assistant Professor, Department of Family and Preventive Medicine, Emory School of Medicine, Atlanta, Georgia

BERNADETTE BAKER, MD
Assistant Professor, Department of Family and Preventive Medicine, Emory School of Medicine, Atlanta, Georgia

ETHAN P. BERG, DO
Assistant Professor, Department of Family and Community Medicine, Southern Illinois University School of Medicine, SIU Decatur Family Medicine Residency, Decatur, Illinois

VICTORIA L. BOGGIANO, MD, MPH
Assistant Professor, Department of Family Medicine, The University of North Carolina at Chapel Hill, Chapel Hill, North Carolina

LIA PIERSON BRUNER, MD
Associate Professor of Family and Community Medicine, Augusta University/University of Georgia Medical Partnership, UGA Health Sciences Campus, Athens, Georgia

LAURA S. CHIU, MD, MPH
Assistant Professor, Department of Medicine, Section of Gastroenterology, Boston University School of Medicine, Boston, Massachusetts

JOHN DAMIANOS, MD
Gastroenterology and Hepatology Fellow, Division of Gastroenterology and Hepatology, Mayo Clinic, Rochester, Minnesota

NEAL D. DHARMADHIKARI, MD
Gastroenterology and Hepatology Fellow, Department of Gastroenterology and Hepatology, Boston University School of Medicine, Boston Medical Center, Boston, Massachusetts

SARA DOSS, MD
Assistant Professor, Loyola University Chicago Stritch School of Medicine, Primary Care, Maywood, Illinois

MOLLY DUFFY, MD
Fellow, Department of Family Medicine, The University of North Carolina at Chapel Hill, Chapel Hill, North Carolina

ALLISON FERRIS, MD, FACP
Chair and Associate Professor of Medicine, Program Director, Internal Medicine Residency Program, Department of Medicine, Charles E. Schmidt College of Medicine, Florida Atlantic University, Boca Raton, Florida

POLINA GAISINSKAYA, MD
Internal Medicine Residency Program, Department of Medicine, Charles E. Schmidt College of Medicine, Graduate Medical Education Consortium, Bethesda Hospital, Boca Raton Regional Hospital, Delray Medical Center, Florida Atlantic University, Boca Raton, Florida

RAVINDRA GANESH, MBBS, MD
Assistant Professor of Medicine, Division of General Internal Medicine, Mayo Clinic, Rochester, Minnesota

C. PRAKASH GYAWALI, MD, MRCP
Professor of Medicine, Division of Gastroenterology, Washington University School of Medicine, St Louis, Missouri

NIDA HAMIDUZZAMAN, MD
Clinical Associate Professor of Medicine, Division of Geriatric, Hospital, Palliative and General Internal Medicine, Keck School of Medicine of USC, Los Angeles, California

EDWARD HURTTE, MD
Division of Gastroenterology, Washington University School of Medicine, St Louis, Missouri

JUHEE C. McDOUGAL, MD
Assistant Professor of Medicine, Boston University School of Medicine, Boston, Massachusetts

KURREN MEHTA, MD
Resident, Department of Medicine, Duke University School of Medicine, Duke University Medical Center, Durham, North Carolina

ASIYA MOHAMMED, MD
Assistant Professor, Department of Family and Community Medicine, Southern Illinois University School of Medicine, SIU Springfield Family Medicine Residency, Springfield, Illinois

MICHAEL MUELLER, MD
Assistant Professor of Medicine, Division of General Internal Medicine, Mayo Clinic, Rochester, Minnesota

NEILANJAN NANDI, MD, FACP
Associate Professor of Clinical Medicine, Division of Gastroenterology and Hepatology, Perelman School of Medicine, University of Pennsylvania, Philadelphia, Pennsylvania

AMIT PATEL, MD
Associate Professor of Medicine, Division of Gastroenterology, Duke University School of Medicine, Durham Veterans Affairs Medical Center, Raleigh, North Carolina

JANAKI PATEL, MD
Assistant Professor of Medicine, Department of Medicine, Ohio State University College of Medicine, Columbus, Ohio

PARVATHI PERUMAREDDI, DO
Associate Professor, Department of Medicine, Florida Atlantic University, Charles E. Schmidt College of Medicine- Florida Atlantic University, Boca Raton, Florida

SETH ANTHONY POLITANO, DO
Associate Professor of Medicine, College of Osteopathic Medicine of the Pacific, Western University of Health Sciences, Pomona, California

KEVIN POLSLEY, MD
Assistant Professor, Loyola University Chicago Stritch School of Medicine, Primary Care, Maywood, Illinois

SIOBHAN PROKSELL, MD
Division of Digestive Health and Liver Disease, Assistant Professor of Clinical Medicine, University of Miami Miller School of Medicine, Miami, Florida

JESSICA ROSENBERG, MD, MHS
Fellow, Department of Gastroenterology, MedStar Georgetown University Hospital, Washington, DC

MEGHA K. SHAH, MD, MSc
Associate Professor, Department of Family and Preventive Medicine, Emory School of Medicine, Atlanta, Georgia

SOFIA D. SHAIKH, MD
Internal Medicine Resident, Department of Internal Medicine, Boston Medical Center, Boston, Massachusetts

ZACHARY J. SHIPP, MD, MS
Assistant Professor, Department of Family and Community Medicine, Southern Illinois University School of Medicine, SIU Decatur Family Medicine Residency, Decatur, Illinois

ORLANDO SOLA, MD, MPH
Formerly, Assistant Professor, Georgetown University, Department of Family Medicine, Washington, DC; Currently, Community clinical practitioner, Baltimore, Maryland

JOHNNY C. TENEGRA, MD, MS
Associate Professor, Department of Family and Community Medicine, Southern Illinois University School of Medicine, SIU Decatur Family Medicine Residency, Decatur, Illinois

EMILY TUERK, MD
Assistant Professor, Loyola University Chicago Stritch School of Medicine, Primary Care, Maywood, Illinois

ADAM VISCONTI, MD, MPH
Assistant Professor, Department of Family Medicine, MedStar Georgetown University, Washington, DC

ANNA MARIE WHITE, MD
Clinical Assistant Professor of Medicine and Pediatrics, University of Pittsburgh School of Medicine, UPMC Shadyside Hospital, Pittsburgh, Pennsylvania

NATALIE WONG, MD
Fellow, Division of Gastroenterology, Duke University School of Medicine, Duke University Medical Center, Durham, North Carolina

JOCELYN YOUNG, DO, MS
United Health Services Hospitals, Johnson City, New York

Contents

Dysphagia is an important clinical symptom that increases in prevalence with age. Both oropharyngeal and esophageal processes can contribute to dysphagia, and these can be differentiated with a careful history. Neuromuscular processes are more prevalent than structural causes in oropharyngeal dysphagia, therefore, investigation should start with a modified barium swallow. In contrast, structural processes dominate in esophageal dysphagia, and endoscopy can offer biopsy and therapy by way of dilation. Manometry is performed for esophageal dysphagia when no structural etiology is found. Specific management of dysphagia is dependent on the etiology and mechanism of dysphagia.

Symptoms potentially attributable to gastroesophageal reflux disease are among those most commonly reported to primary care providers in the outpatient setting. In this review, we discuss clinical approaches to the evaluation and management of these symptoms, including proton pump inhibitor trials as well as specific indications or clinical settings that warrant referral to Gastroenterology specialists.

Peptic ulcer disease is a common cause of epigastric pain typically related to *Helicobacter pylori* infection or NSAID use that can lead to serious consequences including upper GI bleed or perforation if undiagnosed. Diagnostic strategies vary depending on age and treatment is dependent on etiology.

Abnormal liver tests are one of the most common challenges in the primary care setting. Primary care practitioners order these tests for numerous reasons, including investigating abdominal signs and symptoms or suspected alcohol-use disorder, or to determine medication adverse effects.

Evaluation should be guided by both the clinical presentation and the pattern of injury. In this article, we will focus on the epidemiology, pathophysiology, clinical presentation, diagnostic work-up, and management of elevated liver enzymes, with an emphasis on the most common causes of abnormal liver testing.

Diseases of the gallbladder include a spectrum of gallstone diseases (cholelithiasis, cholecystitis, choledocholithiasis, and cholangitis), cysts, polyps, and malignancy. In this review, we present the incidence, risk factors, clinical presentation, diagnosis, and treatment of these various conditions. Importantly, we report when more urgent referral is indicated, as well as red flags that warrant further intervention and/or management.

The pancreas is a vital intra-abdominal organ with dual exocrine and endocrine function. This article provides an overview of several common pancreatic pathologies including pancreatitis, pancreatic cysts, and pancreatic cancer with a focus on clinical presentation as well as initial diagnosis and management.

Crohn disease and ulcerative colitis, the predominant forms of inflammatory bowel disease (IBD), occur in approximately 1% of the population and are typically characterized by chronic diarrhea (with or without bleeding), abdominal pain, and weight loss. The diagnosis is based on history, physical examination, laboratory studies, and endoscopic evaluation. Extraintestinal manifestations may coincide with or precede IBD diagnosis. Treatments have markedly advanced in the past decade, resulting in improved outcomes. IBD, itself, as well as immunosuppressive therapy can increase rates of certain conditions, making collaboration between primary care and gastroenterology imperative for ensuring comprehensive patient care.

Functional gastrointestinal disorders (FGIDs) are an extremely common set of more than 50 disorders characterized by persistent and recurring gastrointestinal symptoms. Most of these patients can be diagnosed and managed by primary care physicians. Treatment includes patient education and reassurance, eliminating triggers, dietary modification, and pharmacologic management. Primary care physicians should consider referral to gastroenterologists when patients exhibit red flag symptoms such as blood in stool, abnormal laboratory findings, involuntary weight loss, age of presentation greater than 50 years, or certain concerning family history.

Gastroenterology

PRIMARY CARE:
CLINICS IN OFFICE PRACTICE

SERIES OF RELATED INTEREST

Medical Clinics (http://www.medical.theclinics.com)
Physician Assistant Clinics (https://www.physicianassistant.theclinics.com)

THE CLINICS ARE AVAILABLE ONLINE!
Access your subscription at:
www.theclinics.com

Foreword

Gut Bacteria: The Good, The Bad, The Necessary

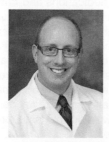

Joel J. Heidelbaugh, MD, FAAFP, FACG
Consulting Editor

Gastrointestinal symptoms and conditions remain a leading concern that drives patients to seek both routine and emergent health care. Over the last decade, much attention has turned toward the role of the microbiome in attempting to define and understand its relationship to many common gastrointestinal disorders. Wolter and colleagues[1] claim that *"by understanding and incorporating the effects of individual dietary components on microbial metabolic output and host physiology, we [can] examine the potential for diet-based therapies for autoimmune disease prevention and treatment."* As many gastrointestinal diseases have an immunologic or genetic basis, it is thought that modulating diet may impact both symptoms and outcomes of disease progression and remission. While we are very early in the game on understanding the intricacies of the microbiome, with each passing year we are learning to appreciate the roles of key bacteria, allowing us to separate out the good, the bad, and the necessary microorganisms that can aid in optimal digestion and health.

What is truly unique about this issue of *Primary Care: Clinics in Office Practice* is that many of the articles take a slightly different approach in presentation of material, often commencing with a gastrointestinal symptom and creating a framework of differential diagnosis to drive therapeutic planning and workup. We trust that this approach will be extremely useful for the primary care provider. Detailed articles on functional bowel disorders provide novel therapeutic strategies for conditions, including irritable bowel syndrome and functional dyspepsia. Other articles provide the current evidence-based guidelines for common gastrointestinal conditions, including gastroesophageal reflux disease, peptic ulcer disease, gastrointestinal bleeding, various forms of dysphagia, and disorders of the gallbladder and pancreas.

The COVID-19 pandemic has wreaked havoc on every possible angle of the health care industry. One commonly impacted facet was the ability to conduct timely

Prim Care Clin Office Pract 50 (2023) xi–xii
https://doi.org/10.1016/j.pop.2023.05.005
0095-4543/23/© 2023 Published by Elsevier Inc.

colorectal cancer screening. To further impact the workforce, guidelines now recommend screening begin at age 45 years. With the rise in obesity and alcohol consumption, we have seen increases in cases of hepatic steatosis as a predominant cause of transaminitis. An article dedicated to highlighting the approach to elevated liver enzymes provides an algorithm approach based upon multiples of the upper limit of normal and concomitant risks. While most primary care providers will not commence pharmacotherapy for treatment of inflammatory bowel disease, it is imperative that we understand how to manage potential adverse effects of medications and comorbid conditions while ensuring appropriate health maintenance provisions.

I would like to congratulate my great colleague, Dr Parvathi Perumareddi, for spearheading a very unique approach to this issue of *Primary Care: Clinics in Office Practice*, which will serve as a salient reference for primary care providers to maximize their care delivery and optimize the appropriateness of referrals to gastroenterology. I offer great thanks to the authors and experts who dedicated their time and energy in writing excellent articles, especially at a time when clinic and professional demands are exceedingly high. Collectively, we hope our readers will find this issue provides key information that is easy to implement in daily practice.

Joel J. Heidelbaugh, MD, FAAFP, FACG
Departments of Family Medicine and Urology
Department of Family Medicine
University of Michigan Medical School
Ann Arbor, MI, USA

Ypsilanti Health Center
200 Arnet Suite 200
Ypsilanti, MI 48198, USA

E-mail address:
jheidel@umich.edu

REFERENCE

1. Wolter M, Grant ET, Boudaud M, et al. Leveraging diet to engineer the gut microbiome. Nat Rev Gastroenterol Hepatol 2021;18(12):885–902.

Preface

From Digestion to Disease and Gut Health: Exploring the Spectrum of the Gastrointestinal System

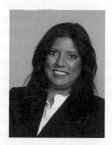

Parvathi Perumareddi, DO
Editor

The gastrointestinal (GI) system consists of multiple organs and is responsible for critical processes from digestion to metabolism. When functioning smoothly, it also assists in absorption of nutrients as well as with multiple other critical processes.

Most people have experienced at least one GI symptom at some point in their lives, and all primary care physicians will encounter one or another GI complaints in their patient visits. GI disease symptoms range from benign to severe, from local or specific to systemic, acute to chronic, and many with the potential to impact quality of life and sometimes longevity. As such, it is vital that the primary care physician be familiar with the presentations of a multitude of GI conditions whose etiologies may not always be apparent at initial presentation. It is equally important to conduct a workup in a methodical and systematic manner to procure a prompt diagnosis for treatment and to be cognizant as to when to refer to GI specialists to avoid complications and/or disease progression.

Where do we begin in diagnosis? We have been taught as primary care physicians to take a complete history and physical of the patient, including inquiring about lifestyle factors for an integrated and holistic approach which can and often does greatly aid in diagnosis; therein lies our starting point. Gathering and analyzing a detailed history encompassing specifics beyond diet and exercise is becoming even more relevant in conjunction with the GI system. Our strong longitudinal relationships with our patients in primary care will no doubt play into this.

The topics included in this edition start with prevalence of the GI conditions, explanation of relevant pathophysiology, discussion of clinical presentation, approach to diagnostic workup, steps in the outline of treatment and prevention where relevant, and finally when to refer to our GI colleagues. As primary care physicians, we anticipate

Prim Care Clin Office Pract 50 (2023) xiii–xv
https://doi.org/10.1016/j.pop.2023.05.004
0095-4543/23/© 2023 Published by Elsevier Inc.

seeing our patients for follow-up, so along with knowledge of these conditions, collaboration with GI or a multidisciplinary approach also becomes crucial for comprehensive and thorough patient care.

If you have ever wondered about the expression "gut feeling" or "gut instinct" it may have more meaning now that research in the past decade has expanded vastly into the area of the gut-brain axis, specifically the microbiome, the community of microorganisms that reside within the digestive tract.

Whereas historically the tendency has been to focus on disease identification and subsequent treatment, we are learning more about this ecosystem in terms of not only its malfunctioning but also how lifestyle modifications can be leveraged to modulate and even prevent disease. This complex system contributes to the normal digestive process and immune function but when there is dysbiosis, numerous malfunctions can occur. Discoveries are showing that other organ systems can be affected by gut flora where pro-inflammatory conditions can potentially arise, leading to severe disease, thus impacting many extra-GI systems, from cardiovascular to neurological and more. While primary care physicians are no stranger to educating patients on therapeutic lifestyle interventions including nutrition and exercise, alcohol and tobacco use, examining these closely and other factors will likely be more critical; what is also becoming more evident is the association of the gut microbiome and its development from birth including the relationship with additional things such as medications (antibiotics), sleep hygiene and stress.

Previously, the thoughts surrounding healthy nutrition focused on calories and macronutrients, including carbohydrates, proteins, and fats, but now there is also information coming forth on specific foods such as fermented ones which contain "good" bacteria and may have a beneficial effect in conjunction with a less processed diet. Studies have shown historically that eastern diets with a variety of plant-based items promoted a "healthier" gut flora but that once folks immigrated to western culture and consumed a diet of more saturated animal fats, processed foods and additives/emulsifiers, the gut bacteria diversity reduced possibly contributing to dysfunction.[1] There may be multiple additional factors that impact gut health starting as early as birth and continuing throughout the life span. Stay tuned to this rapidly advancing field and emerging research on its impact on not only systemic disease management but also on disease prevention.

It is my pleasure to introduce a collection of topics in this gastroenterology edition which we hope will provide the primary care provider with useful diagnostic and management information on a variety of GI conditions with which to deliver the most optimal care to patients. My sincere appreciation goes to the author teams consisting of academic primary care and gastroenterology physicians who assembled the latest information on a variety of important GI subjects in a thorough and detailed fashion, spanning the digestive tract and including current information on colorectal cancer screening.

I would like to express my most genuine thanks to Dr. Joel Heidelbaugh for this wonderful opportunity to serve as guest editor for this edition as well as for his tremendous mentorship and guidance which have been invaluable.

The support from my parents, family, and close friends is what keeps me grounded both personally and professionally, and for that, I remain eternally and humbly grateful. Finally, my dad who exemplifies gratitude, integrity, compassion, kindness and generosity of heart is my role model who inspires me daily not only by his encouragement but also by his example.

As the world evolves post pandemic height into a new era, it is my earnest desire that we take care of and nourish ourselves and others with balance and care which seems fitting with the GI theme.

Parvathi Perumareddi, DO
Department of Medicine
Schmidt College of Medicine
Florida Atlantic University
Boca Raton, FL 33431, USA

E-mail address:
pperumar@health.fau.edu

REFERENCE

1. Vangay P, Johnson AJ, Ward TL, et al. US Immigration Westernizes the Human Gut Microbiome. Cell 2018;175(4): 962-972.e10. doi: 10.1016/j.cell.2018.10.029. PMID: 30388453; PMCID: PMC6498444.

Dysphagia

Edward Hurtte, MD[a], Jocelyn Young, DO, MS[b],
C. Prakash Gyawali, MD, MRCP[a],*

KEYWORDS

- Oropharyngeal dysphagia • Esophageal dysphagia
- Gastroesophageal reflux disease • Achalasia • Aspiration • Stroke

KEY POINTS

- There are two types of dysphagia, oropharyngeal and esophageal, which can be differentiated with a careful history.
- Initial test of choice for evaluation of oropharyngeal dysphagia is a modified barium swallow, as neuromuscular etiologies are more common than structural etiologies.
- Esophageal dysphagia is predominantly caused by structural or mucosal mechanisms, hence endoscopy with biopsy and potential for dilation is most cost effective as the initial test.
- When no structural etiology is identified on endoscopy and/or barium radiography in esophageal dysphagia, a high-resolution manometry study can identify motility disorders.
- Specific management of esophageal dysphagia may require referral to a gastroenterologist.

INTRODUCTION

Dysphagia is the medical term used to describe difficulty swallowing. Dysphagia refers to a subjective sensation of difficulty in the transit of food from mouth to stomach.[1,2] Dysphagia includes difficulty initiating a swallow (termed oropharyngeal dysphagia) as well as the sensation of food being stuck anywhere along the length of the tubular esophagus (termed esophageal dysphagia). Oropharyngeal dysphagia can result from abnormal neural or muscular function of the muscles involved with transfer of food in the mouth, pharynx (back of the throat), and through the upper esophageal sphincter (UES). Diseases that involve the tubular esophagus cause esophageal dysphagia. There are very limited population studies available to determine the prevalence of dysphagia, but the overall prevalence can be estimated from that acquired from a population cohort of over 7000 residents of Olmstead County, MN, where a

a Division of Gastroenterology, Washington University School of Medicine, Campus Box 8124, 660 South Euclid Avenue, St Louis, MO 63110, USA; b United Health Services Hospitals, Johnson City, NY, USA
* Corresponding author.
E-mail address: cprakash@wustl.edu

prevalence of 3% was reported, with a higher prevalence in individuals with heartburn (6%) or regurgitation (11%).[3] The incidence and prevalence of dysphagia increases with age. Prevalence ranges from 5.5% to 8% in persons over the age of 50 years, and is most common in hospitalized and nursing home patients.[4,5] Dysphagia is considered an alarm symptom warranting evaluation as ominous etiologies are possible in addition to benign mechanisms; besides, dysphagia can impact adequate nutrition and can contribute to weight loss.

When a patient presents with dysphagia, it is imperative for the physician to take a careful history to differentiate which type of dysphagia is more likely, as investigation and management differ between oropharyngeal and esophageal dysphagia. Dysphagia needs to be distinguished from odynophagia, defined as pain during swallowing. Odynophagia may arise from infection or inflammation in the throat or esophagus, and rarely from obstructive processes. Dysphagia also needs to be distinguished from globus sensation, defined as a constant sensation of tightness or foreign body sensation at the back of the throat or neck.[2] Globus typically does not impair swallowing and is thought to result from increased perception or hypervigilance in the throat or upper esophagus. In contrast, dysphagia only occurs when attempting to swallow or during the process of swallowing. Globus is occasionally seen in reflux disease; additionally, esophageal mucosal or motor disorders need to be excluded.[6]

Within each oropharyngeal and esophageal dysphagia, there are two broad groups of etiologies, neuromuscular and structural. Neuromuscular causes dominate in oropharyngeal dysphagia, while structural causes are far more common than neuromuscular dysfunction in esophageal dysphagia. The prevalence of each type of dysfunction dictates the order of investigative studies, which is why the tests of choice differ in oropharyngeal versus esophageal dysphagia.

OROPHARYNGEAL DYSPHAGIA

With a careful history and physical examination, the clinician can differentiate oropharyngeal from esophageal dysphagia in 80% to 85% of cases.[7] The prevalence of oropharyngeal dysphagia increases with age due to its relationships to neurologic disorders including cerebrovascular events, movement disorders like Parkinson's disease, and dementia. As many as 70% of individuals are reported to have dysphagia following a cerebrovascular event.[8]

Pathophysiology

The oral phase of swallowing involves breaking down ingested food with chewing, followed by creation of a bolus between the tongue and the palate. The pharyngeal phase requires the oropharyngeal musculature to propel the food bolus into the esophagus through the UES, which opens as part of the pharyngeal phase from relaxation of the cricopharyngeus muscle. The pharyngeal phase also involves laryngeal elevation, and closure of the laryngeal inlet by the epiglottis, to prevent aspiration. The oral or pharyngeal phases of swallowing can be separately compromised in oropharyngeal dysphagia; sometimes both phases can manifest dysfunction.[9] As complex nerve–muscle integration is essential for normal oral and pharyngeal phases of swallowing, etiologies of oropharyngeal dysphagia are commonly neuromuscular rather than structural.[5,7]

Clinical Presentation

Dysphagia is localized to the high neck or back of the throat in oropharyngeal dysphagia. Symptoms are typically reported within 1 second of attempting to swallow.

Patients may complain of coughing, nasal regurgitation, or a choking sensation when attempting to swallow[9] (**Table 1**). Frank aspiration can lead to lower respiratory tract infection, pneumonia, or even a lung abscess, and these could manifest as primary presenting features.[7,10] When the lower cranial nerves are compromised, additional symptoms could include a nasal tone of voice, hoarseness, and drooling of saliva.

When oropharyngeal dysphagia is suspected, physical examination should include inspection of the mouth and oropharynx. In addition, a careful neurologic examination should focus on the motor components of cranial nerves V, VII, IX, X, and XII as well as the sensory components of cranial nerves V, VII, IX, and X, since neuromuscular etiologies are often the cause of oropharyngeal dysphagia (**Table 2**). Neurologic deficits in the upper and lower extremities can also coexist and can provide an important clue to the central localization of neurologic dysfunction in oropharyngeal dysphagia. Examination of the oropharynx includes assessing for adequate saliva.

Structural processes in the nasopharynx and proximal esophagus could include benign webs and strictures. Abnormal cricopharyngeal relaxation can sometimes result in a Zenker's diverticulum in the posterior pharynx. Rarely, neoplasms of the nasopharynx, larynx, or proximal esophagus can result in dysphagia localized to the pharynx or high neck (see **Table 2**).

In addition to globus sensation, xerostomia from reduced saliva production can contribute to the sensation of oropharyngeal dysphagia (**Fig. 1**). Salivary gland hypofunction results in a sensation of difficulty swallowing because of loss of saliva, which is a lubricant for food and a swallow stimulus. Some patients manifest food aversion, which can originate from a fear of perception of dysphagia, especially in patients with anxiety and hypervigilance. Finally, edentulous individuals may report dysphagia from incomplete breakdown of food boluses.

Table 1
Differentiation of oropharyngeal from esophageal dysphagia

	Oropharyngeal Dysphagia	Esophageal Dysphagia
Timing	Within 1 s of swallow initiation	After swallow passes through back of throat
Localization	High neck or throat	Retrosternal area or sternal notch
Associated symptoms	Coughing, aspiration Nasal regurgitation Drooling Hoarseness Nasal tone of voice	Heartburn Chest pain Bland regurgitation of food
Common disorders	Stroke Parkinson's disease Muscular dystrophy Brain stem disorders	GERD Benign strictures Eosinophilic esophagitis
Confounding symptoms/diagnoses	Xerostomia Globus Food aversion	Odynophagia Rumination Globus Food aversion
Test of choice	Videofluoroscopy Modified barium swallow	Upper endoscopy
Secondary tests	Fiberoptic laryngoscopy CT scan of head and neck Blood tests for myositis, myasthenia	Barium swallow High-resolution manometry

Table 2	
Etiology of oropharyngeal dysphagia	
Neuromuscular	Cerebrovascular accident
	Parkinson's disease
	Amyotrophic lateral sclerosis
	Poliomyelitis
	Brain stem disorders
	Brain tumors
	Polymyositis, dermatomyositis
	Muscular dystrophy
	Myasthenia gravis
	Abnormal upper esophageal sphincter
Structural	Inflammation: pharyngitis
	Radiation-related strictures
	Zenker's diverticulum
	Benign webs and strictures
	Cervical hyperostosis
	Oral, pharyngeal, and laryngeal cancer
	Thyromegaly

Diagnostic Testing

When oropharyngeal dysphagia is suspected, the initial test of choice is video fluoro-scopic contrast radiography, also termed modified barium swallow (MBS), which can be ordered by the primary care physician (see **Fig. 1**). MBS provides lateral and ante-roposterior views of the oral and pharyngeal phases of swallowing, using boluses of varying consistency (thin liquid, thick liquid, semisolid, solid). In addition to identifying neuromuscular dysfunction, MBS determines oropharyngeal clearance of food, and elucidates structural abnormalities when present, including a Zenker's diverticulum. During the procedure, a speech pathologist instructs the patient on neck position and maneuvers that are most likely to result adequate oropharyngeal clearance into the esophagus without aspiration. Thus, MBS is utilized in identifying the location and severity of oropharyngeal neuromuscular dysfunction, and determining the

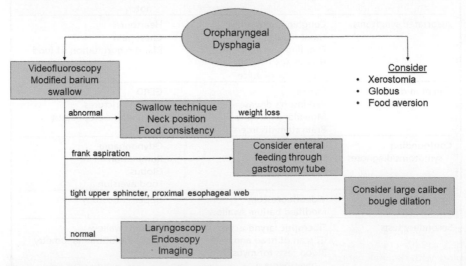

Fig. 1. Algorithm for evaluation of oropharyngeal dysphagia.

influence of bolus consistency and posture on bolus clearance or aspiration risk (**Fig. 2**). Specific swallow therapies can be recommended based on MBS findings, including bypassing the oropharynx completely using enteral feeding when aspiration risk is high.

MBS can be complemented by high-resolution manometry (HRM) combined with stationary impedance, which can assess pharyngeal, upper sphincter, and proximal esophageal function in addition to distal esophageal motor physiology and pathophysiology[11]; however, this remains a research tool in most esophageal centers. Trans nasal fiberoptic laryngoscopy or fiberoptic endoscopic examination of swallowing can determine presence of pharyngeal pooling during test swallows, as well as structural processes in the nasopharynx, oropharynx, and larynx. Upper endoscopy visualizes the oropharyngeal and esophageal mucosa and can identify additional mucosal and structural processes including webs, strictures, and diverticula including Zenker's diverticulum. Cross-sectional imaging (CT or MRI scans) can evaluate soft tissues in the head and neck; these tests are also utilized for evaluation of space occupying lesions or other abnormalities in the brain, brain stem, cervical spinal cord, and cranial nerves.

Skeletal muscle dysfunction can contribute to oropharyngeal dysphagia in rare instances. These disorders include autoimmune myositides (polymyalgia rheumatica, polymyositis, dermatomyositis, and other idiopathic myositides), muscular dystrophy, and myasthenia gravis. In addition to inflammatory markers (erythrocyte sedimentation rate [ESR], C reactive protein [CRP]), muscle enzymes can be elevated (creatine kinase, aldolase). Specific autoimmune markers are available for some of these disorders of skeletal muscle.

Management

Management of oropharyngeal dysphagia necessitates a multidisciplinary team approach that includes the primary care physician, speech pathologist, nutritionist, gastroenterologist, neurologist, and sometimes rheumatologist. When specific abnormalities are found, these are targeted. Examples of specific management include

- Endoscopic dilation for webs and strictures
- Diverticulectomy for Zenker's diverticulum, and
- Anti-inflammatory agents or steroids for myositides.

However, most of the central and peripheral neurologic causes may not be amenable to specific treatment, and management of individual symptoms, food transit, and nutrition will be of key importance in these instances.

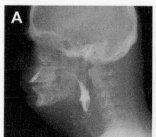 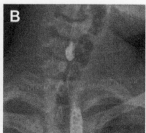 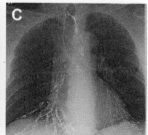

Fig. 2. Images from videofluoroscopy performed for oropharyngeal dysphagia. (*A*). Pharyngeal residue due to a poorly relaxing cricopharyngeus muscle. (*B*). A small Zenker's diverticulum with retained contrast in the posterior pharynx. (*C*). Aspiration of barium resulting in bronchial opacification.

The goals of management include minimizing the risk of aspiration and maintaining adequate nutrition. When aspiration risk is not deemed to be high, neck positioning and altering food consistency can be of value in achieving management goals (see **Fig. 1**). Speech pathologists can assist with specific food consistency recommendations, optimal positioning, and strengthening exercises. If maintaining adequate nutrition becomes challenging, or if aspiration risk is high, enteral feeding on a temporary or permanent basis may be necessary.

ESOPHAGEAL DYSPHAGIA

Esophageal dysphagia refers to dysphagia arising from disruption of bolus transit within the tubular esophagus after the bolus has traversed the UES. Structural causes are far more frequent than disorders involving nerves or muscles (**Table 3**). Therefore, luminal narrowing of the esophagus (strictures), mucosal inflammation from reflux disease or other inflammatory disorders, tumors within the esophagus, and compression of the lumen from intramural or extrinsic causes, and rarely, neoplasms of the esophagus can contribute to esophageal dysphagia. Benign strictures are often encountered, most often related to gastroesophageal reflux. Idiopathic benign strictures such as the Schatzki ring at the squamocolumnar junction can cause intermittent solid food dysphagia. Mucosal infiltration of eosinophils (eosinophilic esophagitis) can result in compromise to the esophageal lumen from mucosal inflammation, wall stiffness, and fibrosis. Eosinophilic esophagitis is thought to be triggered by dietary and/or environmental allergens in predisposed individuals. Pill induced inflammation can also result in strictures with the most common culprits being

- Nonsteroidal anti-inflammatory agents
- Doxycycline
- Alendronate
- Quinine, and
- Potassium supplements

Pill esophagitis can also be a consequence of other types of strictures, or motor obstruction.

Table 3	
Etiology of esophageal dysphagia	
Structural	Benign webs and strictures
	Gastroesophageal reflux disease
	Eosinophilic esophagitis
	Esophageal cancer
	Past esophageal surgery (fundoplication)
	Paraesophageal hernia
	Lichen planus
	Extrinsic compression
	Caustic injury
	Radiation-induced strictures
	Vascular compression (dysphagia lusoria)
Neuromuscular	Achalasia spectrum disorders
	Distal esophageal spasm
	Hypercontractile esophagus (Jackhammer)
	Chagas disease
	Scleroderma, mixed connective tissue disease

Less common are disorders involving esophageal neuromuscular function. The most consequential of these disorders is achalasia, where the lower esophageal sphincter (LES) fails to relax during swallowing, from abnormal esophageal inhibitory nerve function. This is typically associated with absent or abnormal peristalsis in the esophageal body proximal to the esophagus. Less frequently, the esophageal smooth muscle demonstrates exaggerated or premature contraction, loosely termed esophageal spastic disorders. Advanced motor disorders like achalasia are irreversible, and treatment typically involves disruption or surgical incision of the LES to relieve the obstruction. Some forms of esophageal motor obstruction can be a consequence of opioid use, and the resulting motor pattern can mimic some forms of achalasia. Other motor disorders manifest weakness of both esophageal body smooth muscle as well as the LES. In extreme situations, the muscle generates no force and is unable to generate peristalsis. Although dysphagia may be a symptom with these hypomotility disorders, there is no true obstruction, and the esophagus can clear its contents with the help of gravity as long as the patient eats while upright. Reflux is a more important consequence, and postural measures are typically recommended to avoid reflux-induced complications.

Clinical Presentation

With esophageal dysphagia, food may be swallowed normally, but may get stuck in the neck or chest. Localization of esophageal dysphagia can vary depending on the site of the abnormality causing dysphagia. Even though the abnormality may be at the bottom end of the esophagus, the sensation of food being stuck may be felt higher up in the chest or even in the neck region (see **Table 1**). However, it is important to note that esophageal dysphagia never localizes lower than the site of obstruction. Sometimes, swallowed food may be regurgitated back into the mouth when it may taste like the food just eaten. This should be differentiated from reflux of gastric content, which is often sour and bitter.

With structural disorders, dysphagia is initially reported with solids and not with liquids. With tight obstructions, difficulty with liquids can develop, but difficulty is typically worse with solids, especially dry solids and pills. Symptoms of reflux disease such as heartburn may coexist, since reflux is the most common cause of esophageal strictures causing dysphagia. Rarely, a food bolus may block the lumen of the esophagus, termed food impaction. This is seen with tight strictures, and especially with eosinophilic esophagitis. Food impaction can manifest as a total inability to swallow, including liquids, and requires urgent endoscopy for dis-impaction of the food bolus. In contrast,

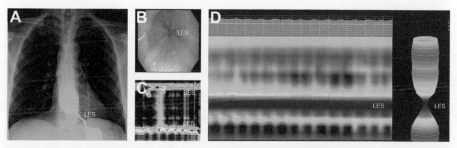

Fig. 3. Test results in a patient with achalasia. (*A*). Barium swallow demonstrating a dilated esophagus with a tapered distal esophagus indicating a closed LES. (*B*). Endoscopic image showing a tight and puckered LES. (*C*). HRM Clouse plot showing no esophageal body peristalsis, and no relaxation of the LES with swallows. (*D*). Two images from a FLIP study showing a tight, non-relaxing LES.

neuromuscular dysfunction such as achalasia and motor disorders result in dysphagia to both solids and liquids. These symptoms slowly develop over time in achalasia, where relaxation of the LES during swallowing is incomplete (**Fig. 3**). Therefore, the condition may be difficult to diagnose at the outset, but symptoms can become severe enough to result in weight loss. Sometimes, achalasia-like disorders develop from cancers at the esophagogastric junction, termed pseudo-achalasia, where symptoms similar to achalasia develop over a short period of time, and with profound weight loss. Neuromuscular disorders of the esophagus, particularly spastic disorders and some forms of achalasia, may also be associated with atypical chest pain; in these instances, it is important to rule out a cardiac cause of chest pain before attributing this symptom to the esophagus.

Diagnosis

A careful history can differentiate esophageal dysphagia from oropharyngeal dysphagia. The patient typically reports food being stuck somewhere between the neck and the epigastrium, for varying periods of time before the food passes (see **Table 1**). There may be a regurgitation of the ingested food, and the patient may sometimes induce regurgitation for relief. Some patients develop pain or discomfort when the food is stuck and may report pain during eating as their primary symptom.

As strictures and other structural or mucosal processes are the most frequent mechanisms of esophageal dysphagia, evaluation requires consideration of gastroesophageal reflux disease (GERD) in the etiology.[11] Dysphagia is an alarm symptom, especially in patients with GERD symptoms, and indicates a need for invasive evaluation for strictures, esophagitis, and other complications of GERD, all of which can cause dysphagia.[12,13] Eosinophilic esophagitis (EoE) is an important differential diagnosis for a structural cause of esophageal dysphagia.[14] Consequently, upper endoscopy is a common investigative procedure performed in the setting of alarm symptoms (**Fig. 4**).

Endoscopy has several advantages over barium radiography in the evaluation of esophageal dysphagia. Endoscopy not only identifies reflux-induced (peptic)

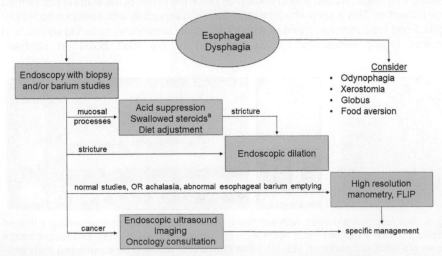

Fig. 4. Algorithm for evaluation of esophageal dysphagia.[a]If eosinophilic esophagitis is diagnosed.

strictures that cause dysphagia, but can also provide management using balloon or bougie dilators during the same procedure.[12] Peptic strictures are seen more often in older patients, patients with long-standing untreated reflux symptoms, and those with a hiatus hernia, although the incidence is decreasing with the widespread use of proton pump inhibitors (PPIs).[15] Endoscopy also provides the characterization of esophageal mucosal injury (**Fig. 5**), seen as longitudinal or circumferential erosions in the distal esophageal mucosa, which can result in dysphagia even without the presence of strictures or other processes.[16] The Los Angeles (LA) Classification descriptively characterizes reflux esophagitis into four grades from A through D. Using the LA grading system, patients with LA Grades C or D esophagitis are more likely to present with dysphagia (43%), compared to LA Grades A or B (43% vs 36%, P <.001).[16] About 10% to 15% of patients with chronic GERD can develop Barrett's esophagus, where metaplastic columnar mucosa replaces the normal squamous esophageal mucosa in the distal esophagus. Barrett's esophagus is a risk factor for esophageal adenocarcinoma, which can cause luminal compromise and dysphagia. Therefore, there is a role for endoscopic screening of patients with long-standing GERD, as identification and ablation of dysplasia within Barrett's esophagus can reduce the incidence of esophageal adenocarcinoma. In this context, Caucasian men aged >50 years, with obesity, smoking, and a family history of esophageal cancer carry the highest risk for Barrett's esophagus and esophageal adenocarcinoma.[17,18] Endoscopy also serves to diagnose esophageal cancer when present and is part of the staging of cancer (using endoscopic ultrasound), and the palliation of cancer (using stents).

An important condition associated with dysphagia and food bolus impaction is eosinophilic esophagitis (EoE),[19] symptoms of which can overlap with GERD. Diagnosis of EoE is contingent on the finding of eosinophilia (>15 eosinophils per high power field) on esophageal biopsies, which makes endoscopy the test of choice in the evaluation of esophageal dysphagia as biopsies can be taken (see **Fig. 5**).

Barium radiography is very sensitive for the identification of subtle strictures and rings in the esophagus, particularly when a standard barium swallow is combined with a 13 mm barium pill swallow, or a marshmallow or cookie impregnated with barium.[20] Barium studies can also accurately define hiatus hernias, particularly paraoesophageal hernias, as these can contribute to dysphagia. A timed upright barium study, where x-rays are taken in the upright position 1 minute and 5 minutes following administration of 8 oz of semiliquid barium, can demonstrate if esophageal emptying is compromised from obstruction at the esophagogastric junction. Barium studies, therefore, complement endoscopy and alternate evaluation methods such as

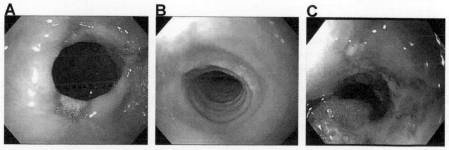

Fig. 5. Endoscopic images of findings in patients with esophageal dysphagia. (*A*). Peptic stricture in the distal esophagus, with esophagitis. (*B*). Corrugated, ringed esophagus in eosinophilic esophagitis. (*C*). Growth protruding into the lumen in esophageal cancer.

manometry and functional lumen imaging probe (FLIP) in the evaluation of esophageal dysphagia.

When no structural etiology is found in the evaluation of esophageal dysphagia, or if endoscopy and/or barium findings lead to suspicion of a motility disorder, an esophageal manometry can be performed.[20] HRM is the current standard, where a catheter with multiple circumferential high sensitivity sensors is introduced through an anesthetized nostril into the esophagus and positioned with a few sensors located in the stomach. Topographic images of esophageal peristalsis and sphincter function can be displayed and interrogated with software tools. HRM is the gold standard for the diagnosis of motility disorders, particularly achalasia, using the Chicago Classification v4.0, a hierarchical algorithm that defines criteria for diagnosis.[21] The combination of impedance with HRM, termed high-resolution impedance manometry can allow the bolus to be visualized, and can demonstrate abnormal bolus transit if present.

The newest esophageal investigative procedure is FLIP.[22] This incorporates impedance methodology, with pairs of electrodes on a catheter encased in a compliant balloon. The catheter is placed through the mouth after sedated upper endoscopy and positioned with the balloon straddling the esophagogastric junction. With volumetric distension of the balloon using an electrolyte-containing fluid, cross-sectional area, and lumen diameter can be measured throughout the esophagus and across the esophagogastric junction. The relationship between cross-sectional area and distending pressure (measured using a sensor incorporated into the catheter) is depicted as the distensibility index (DI).[22] Low DI (combined with low opening diameter) is seen with abnormal LES relaxation associated with achalasia spectrum disorders. Normal DI with low diameter defines a structural process such as a stricture, while both DI and diameter are within normal range if there is no obstructive element. Topographic plots of diameter against time across the evaluated segment of the esophagus can demonstrate esophageal secondary peristalsis, which can provide clues to esophageal body motor function.

Thus, endoscopy, barium radiography, HRM, and FLIP provide complementary information in the evaluation of dysphagia.

If no structural or motor abnormalities are identified on esophageal testing, the sensation of dysphagia could be perceptive from increased visceral sensation, and functional dysphagia can be diagnosed.[2] Psychiatric co-morbidities such as anxiety, depression, and somatoform disorders are common among patients with functional gastrointestinal disorders. Dysphagia is the least common functional esophageal disorder, accounting for only 2.4% of adults presenting with dysphagia in a large tertiary care center,[23] and requires exclusion of esophageal mucosal processes including eosinophilic esophagitis, gastroesophageal reflux disease, and major motor disorders.[2]

Treatment

For the most part, treatment of dysphagia depends on the cause. Some general measures that are often recommended include changing the consistency of food, as soft food items or liquids may traverse a narrowed esophageal lumen better than hard, dry solids. Patients are advised to eat in the upright position and push solids down with sips of fluid when necessary. Standing up and/or raising arms above the head can straighten the esophagus and may allow intrathoracic pressure with breathing to compress the esophagus and empty contents into the stomach. When nutrition is compromised, the esophagus may need to be bypassed in favor of enteral feeding into the stomach or small intestine through feeding tubes.

As strictures are often encountered as a mechanism for esophageal dysphagia, endoscopic therapy can be provided at the index endoscopy, using either through-the-scope balloon dilators, or bougies passed either over a guide wire placed during endoscopy (Savary-Guillard dilators) or passed blind (Maloney dilators).[24] When long, narrow strictures are encountered, fluoroscopy can provide a road map for placement of a guide wire, especially when the stricture is not traversed with the endoscope. Rarely, stents are placed for the management of refractory strictures, but these need to be anchored in place when used for benign strictures. Perforation rates are higher with malignant obstruction, and are rare with benign processes like strictures.[25]

Acid suppression using a PPI is typically part of the management, as most strictures are related to reflux disease.[26] Strictures and luminal narrowing can also be seen with EoE, where management starts with either PPI or topical steroid, sometimes complemented with the elimination of some or all the most common food items associated with EoE (milk, gluten, tree nuts, seafood, eggs, soy).[27,28] Recently, dupilumab has been approved by the Food and Drug Administration (FDA) for the management of EoE at a dose of 300 mg weekly administered subcutaneously.[29] Treatment of inflammation first using these measures makes endoscopic dilation much more effective in EoE. When endoscopic dilation is required, chest pain is the most frequent adverse effect requiring analgesics, and perforation is rare.

Among other benign etiologies, pill esophagitis is treated with discontinuation of the offending medication, and infectious esophagitis is treated with specific agents directed at the infectious agent.

Motility disorders with abnormal LES relaxation such as achalasia require disruption or surgical incision of the LES for durable symptom relief. This can be achieved through forceful pneumatic or hydraulic dilation, myotomy of the LES through the abdominal route (laparoscopic Heller myotomy), or myotomy through the esophageal route (per oral endoscopic myotomy or POEM).[30] Reflux can be a consequence and may require management with PPI. Temporary benefit can be achieved with the injection of botulinum toxin into the LES during endoscopy, and this can be used as a bridge to durable management, or as the primary management option when the patient is a poor candidate for invasive management. Rarely, esophagectomy is performed for a massively dilated esophagus. Feeding past the esophagus using a gastrostomy tube is an alternative.

Malignant obstruction of the esophagus requires targeted management that can include neoadjuvant chemoradiation and/or surgical resection with a gastric pull-up. Palliation of inoperable tumors may include placement of a stent to keep the esophageal lumen open.

When to Refer

The initial evaluation of oropharyngeal dysphagia can be initiated by the primary care provider, who may order MBS, and have the patient follow instructions provided by the speech pathologist who participates in the MBS. Consultation with a neurologist may be useful when neuromuscular etiologies are considered. Consultation with an ear-nose-throat specialist can help rule out structural processes in the pharynx and larynx. A gastroenterologist can help with the placement of a gastrostomy tube for enteral feeding in instances where aspiration risk is high, or when nutrition is compromised. Endoscopic empiric large-caliber bougie dilation is sometimes performed for dysphagia localized to the high neck where evaluation is negative.

Esophageal dysphagia typically requires referral to a gastroenterologist, especially if symptoms persist despite trials of acid suppression with a PPI, because endoscopy is an alarm symptom needing invasive investigation. Endoscopy, with the potential for biopsy and endoscopic dilation, becomes more cost effective than a barium radiograph, as an abnormal finding on barium studies will require an endoscopy for biopsy and management.

SUMMARY

A thorough history is a vital starting point in the evaluation of dysphagia, as the history can differentiate oropharyngeal from esophageal dysphagia. Mechanisms and etiologies vary widely between oropharyngeal and esophageal dysphagia. As neuromuscular causes dominate, evaluation of oropharyngeal dysphagia starts with MBS. In contrast, as structural mechanisms are found more often than neuromuscular dysfunction in esophageal dysphagia, an upper endoscopy offers both diagnosis and therapeutic intervention, as dilation can be performed at index endoscopy. Once the etiology is determined, specific management can be offered targeting the cause of dysphagia, if this is available.

CLINICS CARE POINTS

- When evaluating a patient with dysphagia, take a careful history to differentiate oropharyngeal dysphagia from esophageal dysphagia
- When investigating oropharyngeal dysphagia, request an MBS to optimize swallow technique and food consistency, and to evaluate for aspiration
- When treating oropharyngeal dysphagia with significant aspiration or weight loss, consider enteral feeding through a gastrostomy tube
- When a patient has esophageal dysphagia, refer for upper endoscopy before empiric acid suppression for diagnosis of the mechanism of dysphagia, and potential therapy
- When a patient presents with a history of food impaction, consider eosinophilic esophagitis as a diagnostic possibility
- When a patient with intermittent solid food dysphagia has normal upper endoscopy with biopsies, consider a barium swallow including a barium pill swallow to identify subtle strictures or other mechanical processes
- When esophageal dysphagia is not explained by endoscopy and/or barium radiography, request an esophageal HRM to identify or rule out achalasia spectrum disorders

DISCLOSURES

No conflicts of interest exist. No funding was obtained. E. Hurtte: no disclosures; J. Young: no disclosures; C.P. Gyawali: Medtronic, Ardelyx, Dexcel Pharma.

REFERENCES

1. Spechler SJ. AGA technical review on treatment of patients with dysphagia caused by benign disorders of the distal esophagus. Gastroenterology 1999; 117(1):233–54.
2. Aziz Q, Fass R, Gyawali CP, et al. Functional Esophageal Disorders. Gastroenterology 2016;150:1368–79.
3. Sawada A, Guzman M, Nikaki K, et al. Identification of Different Phenotypes of Esophageal Reflux Hypersensitivity and Implications for Treatment. Clin Gastroenterol Hepatol 2021;19(4):690–698 e2.

4. Lindgren S, Janzon L. Prevalence of swallowing complaints and clinical findings among 50-79-year-old men and women in an urban population. Dysphagia 1991; 6(4):187–92.
5. Adkins C, Takakura W, Spiegel BMR, et al. Prevalence and Characteristics of Dysphagia Based on a Population-Based Survey. Clin Gastroenterol Hepatol 2020;18(9):1970–1979 e2.
6. Zerbib F, Rommel N, Pandolfino J, et al. ESNM/ANMS Review. Diagnosis and management of globus sensation: A clinical challenge. Neuro Gastroenterol Motil 2020;32(9):e13850.
7. Spicker MR. Evaluating dysphagia. Am Fam Physician 2000;61(12):3639–48.
8. Martino R, Beaton D, Diamant NE. Perceptions of psychological issues related to dysphagia differ in acute and chronic patients. Dysphagia 2010;25(1):26–34.
9. Rommel N, Hamdy S. Oropharyngeal dysphagia: manifestations and diagnosis. Nat Rev Gastroenterol Hepatol 2016;13(1):49–59.
10. Johnston BT. Oesophageal dysphagia: a stepwise approach to diagnosis and management. Lancet Gastroenterol Hepatol 2017;2(8):604–9.
11. Triggs J, Pandolfino J. Recent advances in dysphagia management. F1000Res 2019;8. https://doi.org/10.12688/f1000research.18900.1.
12. Katz PO, Gerson LB, Vela MF. Guidelines for the diagnosis and management of gastroesophageal reflux disease. Am J Gastroenterol 2013;108(3):308–28, quiz 29.
13. Shaheen NJ, Weinberg DS, Denberg TD, et al. Upper endoscopy for gastro-esophageal reflux disease: best practice advice from the clinical guidelines committee of the American College of Physicians. Annals of internal medicine 2012; 157(11):808–16.
14. Savarino E, Bredenoord AJ, Fox M, et al. Expert consensus document: Advances in the physiological assessment and diagnosis of GERD. Nat Rev Gastroenterol Hepatol 2017;14(11):665–76.
15. Cho SY, Choung RS, Saito YA, et al. Prevalence and risk factors for dysphagia: a USA community study. Neuro Gastroenterol Motil 2015;27(2):212–9.
16. Vakil NB, Traxler B, Levine D. Dysphagia in patients with erosive esophagitis: prevalence, severity, and response to proton pump inhibitor treatment. Clin Gastroenterol Hepatol 2004;2(8):665–8.
17. Spechler SJ, Sharma P, Souza RF, et al. American Gastroenterological Association technical review on the management of Barrett's esophagus. Gastroenterology 2011;140(3):e18–52, quiz e13.
18. Shaheen NJ, Falk GW, Iyer PG, et al. ACG Clinical Guideline: Diagnosis and Management of Barrett's Esophagus. Am J Gastroenterol 2016;111(1):30–50, quiz 1.
19. Dellon ES, Hirano I. Epidemiology and Natural History of Eosinophilic Esophagitis. Gastroenterology 2018;154(2):319–332 e3.
20. Gyawali CP, Carlson DA, Chen JW, et al. ACG Clinical Guidelines: Clinical Use of Esophageal Physiologic Testing. Am J Gastroenterol 2020;115(9):1412–28.
21. Yadlapati R, Kahrilas PJ, Fox MR, et al. Esophageal motility disorders on high-resolution manometry: Chicago classification version 4.0((c)). Neuro Gastroenterol Motil 2021;33(1):e14058.
22. Savarino E, di Pietro M, Bredenoord AJ, et al. Use of the Functional Lumen Imaging Probe in Clinical Esophagology. Am J Gastroenterol 2020;115(11):1786–96.
23. Bill J, Rajagopal S, Kushnir V, et al. Diagnostic yield in the evaluation of dysphagia: experience at a single tertiary care center. Dis Esophagus 2018; 31(6). https://doi.org/10.1093/dote/doy013.

24. Ravich WJ. Endoscopic Management of Benign Esophageal Strictures. Curr Gastroenterol Rep 2017;19(10):50.
25. Grooteman KV, Wong Kee, Song LM, Vleggaar FP, et al. Non-adherence to the rule of 3 does not increase the risk of adverse events in esophageal dilation. Gastrointest Endosc 2017;85(2):332–337 e1.
26. Gyawali CP, Fass R. Management of Gastroesophageal Reflux Disease. Gastroenterology 2018;154(2):302–18.
27. Dellon ES, Jensen ET, Martin CF, et al. Prevalence of Eosinophilic Esophagitis in the United States. Clin Gastroenterol Hepatol 2013;12(4):589–96.e1.
28. Dellon ES, Liacouras CA, Molina-Infante J, et al. Updated International Consensus Diagnostic Criteria for Eosinophilic Esophagitis: Proceedings of the AGREE Conference. Gastroenterology 2018;155(4):1022–1033 e10.
29. Hirano I, Dellon ES, Hamilton JD, et al. Efficacy of Dupilumab in a Phase 2 Randomized Trial of Adults With Active Eosinophilic Esophagitis. Gastroenterology 2020;158(1):111–122 e10.
30. Savarino E, Bhatia S, Roman S, et al. Achalasia. Nat Rev Dis Primers 2022; 8(1):28.

Gastroesophageal Reflux Disease

Janaki Patel, MD[a], Natalie Wong, MD[b], Kurren Mehta, MD[c], Amit Patel, MD[d,e],*

KEYWORDS

- Gastroesophageal reflux disease • Heartburn • Regurgitation
- Proton pump inhibitor • Ambulatory reflux monitoring • Esophageal function testing
- High-resolution manometry

KEY POINTS

- The presence of alarm features (such as dysphagia, weight loss, gastrointestinal bleeding, anemia, persistent vomiting) should warrant endoscopic evaluation among patients with suspected gastroesophageal reflux disease (GERD).
- In the setting of appropriate indications for their use, the proven benefits of proton pump inhibitors outweigh potential theoretical risks raised by observational data.
- Indications for screening for Barrett's esophagus (BE) include chronic GERD symptoms and at least three additional risk factors for BE (male, age >50 years, White race, tobacco use, obesity, family history of esophageal adenocarcinoma).
- Patients with isolated extra-esophageal symptoms warrant directed work-up, which may include referral to otorhinolaryngology (Ear, Nose, and Throat), pulmonary, and/or allergy specialists as appropriate based on the clinical presentation.

INTRODUCTION

Symptoms potentially attributable to gastroesophageal reflux disease (GERD) represent common indications for presentation to primary care providers in clinical practice. These symptoms may be typical (heartburn or regurgitation) or atypical (ie, chest pain or cough) in nature. Although these symptoms may stem from GERD and accordingly respond to appropriate treatments, other non-GERD processes may be responsible for contributing to these symptoms.[1] These may include mucosal or structural processes (such as eosinophilic or infectious esophagitis, hiatus hernia, malignancy), esophageal motor disorders (such as achalasia or hypercontractility), behavioral

[a] Department of Medicine, Ohio State University College of Medicine, 410 West 10th Avenue, Columbus, OH 43210, USA; [b] Division of Gastroenterology, Duke University School of Medicine, Duke University Medical Center, Box 3913, Durham, NC 27710, USA; [c] Department of Medicine, Duke University School of Medicine, Duke University Medical Center, Box 3913, Durham, NC 27710, USA; [d] Division of Gastroenterology, Duke University School of Medicine, 10207 Cerny Street, Suite 200, Raleigh, NC 27617, USA; [e] Division of Gastroenterology, Durham Veterans Affairs Medical Center
* Corresponding author. Division of Gastroenterology, Duke University School of Medicine, 10207 Cerny Street, Suite 200, Raleigh, NC 27617.
E-mail address: Amit.patel@duke.edu

Prim Care Clin Office Pract 50 (2023) 339–350
https://doi.org/10.1016/j.pop.2023.03.002
0095-4543/23/Published by Elsevier Inc.
primarycare.theclinics.com

disorders (such as rumination syndrome or supragastric belching), disorders of gut–brain interaction (such as functional heartburn), or non-esophageal disorders (such as cardiac, pulmonary, or ENT processes).[2]

A careful history and physical exam are paramount in the primary care setting, and empiric proton pump inhibitor (PPI) trials represent a pragmatic and cost-effective diagnostic strategy, particularly for typical symptoms of heartburn and/or regurgitation in the absence of alarm symptoms.[3–5] However, in other clinical settings, such as if alarm features are present, or if symptoms persist despite an appropriate PPI trial, referral to gastroenterology is appropriate for further evaluation and diagnostic testing.[3] Here, we discuss approaches to these potential GERD symptoms in the primary care setting and indications for referral to gastroenterology (**Fig. 1**).

Prevalence

GERD has an immense—and increasing—global burden. A systematic analysis of the Global Burden of Disease Study data revealed estimates ranges of age-standardized GERD prevalence at 4408 to 14,035 per 100,000 population.[6] Systematic review analysis of population-based studies estimates GERD prevalence at 18% to 28% in North America.[7] Data-based estimates suggest more than 4.7 million visits for GERD or reflux esophagitis provider diagnoses annually in the United States.[8]

Pathophysiology

At its core, GERD is characterized by the retrograde flow (reflux) of gastric contents into the esophagus leading to bothersome symptoms and/or mucosal injury or

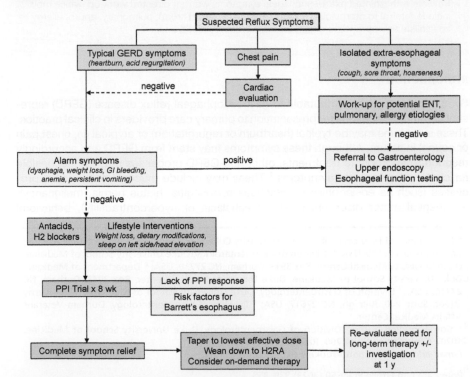

Fig. 1. Primary care clinical algorithm for the evaluation and management of patients with suspected gastroesophageal reflux disease symptoms.

complications.[9] Various mechanisms can contribute to GERD, such as the acidity and burden of refluxate, the proximal extent of refluxate, impaired esophageal peristalsis and/or clearance of refluxate, lower esophageal sphincter dysfunction, disruption of the gastroesophageal junction, increased gastric pressures, reduced gastric emptying, esophageal hypersensitivity, and cognitive hypervigilance.[4,10]

Clinical Presentation

Patients often present to primary care clinics reporting symptoms suspicious for or consistent with GERD. These can include symptoms typical for GERD (heartburn and/or regurgitation) as well as atypical for GERD (ie, chest pain, cough). These symptoms are so commonly experienced that patients often self-diagnose GERD. Moreover, as multiple treatment options are available over the counter, patients may also initiate treatments themselves before presentation to their primary care provider. Therefore, as a primary care provider, it is imperative to appropriately characterize symptoms and understand potential indications for further diagnosis, management, and referral.[11]

Heartburn and regurgitation are characterized as *typical* GERD symptoms. The most common symptom of GERD is considered heartburn, typically described by patients as a substernal burning sensation, rising from the epigastrium, perhaps noted after meals. They may also report regurgitation, typically described as a rising of gastric contents toward the mouth, with or without an associated acidic or bitter taste.

Potential extra-esophageal symptoms of GERD can be challenging to identify and characterize as they may be more non-specific and even overlap. These may be reported by patients as

- Cough
- Sore throat
- Throat clearing
- Laryngitis
- Globus, and/or
- Hoarseness

Particularly when isolated (ie, in the absence of typical GERD symptoms), these symptoms have poor sensitivity and specificity for GERD, and referral to otorhinolaryngology (ENT), pulmonary, and/or allergy specialists is often appropriate based on the clinical presentation. In these settings, there is less enthusiasm for and effectiveness of prolonged treatment with PPIs, as this can delay diagnosis, and gastroenterology referral with associated diagnostic testing may be considered.[3]

Because of the location of the esophagus, patients with GERD may present with chest pain, which can be indistinguishable from the pain associated with cardiac etiologies. Because chest pain has a broad differential diagnosis that includes life-threatening cardiovascular conditions, it is imperative for primary care providers to first rule out such diseases. If heart disease has been adequately excluded, then a PPI trial for typical reflux symptoms as discussed below may be appropriate before referral to gastroenterology for further evaluation (with endoscopy, manometry, and/or ambulatory reflux monitoring as indicated). Although PPI trials have been utilized in such patients with noncardiac chest pain, symptom improvement is typically associated with the presence of abnormal endoscopy and/or reflux monitoring findings.

Although patients with typical GERD symptoms may be empirically treated with PPI trials, it is critical to refer patients with alarm symptoms to gastroenterology and/or upper endoscopy promptly. Potential alarm features can include evidence of gastrointestinal bleeding, iron deficiency anemia, unexplained weight loss, dysphagia,

> **Box 1**
> **Potential alarm symptoms in patients with suspected gastroesophageal reflux disease to prompt gastroenterology referral and endoscopic evaluation**
>
> Potential Alarm Features to Prompt Gastroenterology Referral for Endoscopy
> - Dysphagia or odynophagia
> - Unintentional weight loss
> - Gastrointestinal bleeding
> - Anemia
> - Persistent vomiting
>
> *Data from* Katz PO, Dunbar KB, Schnoll-Sussman FH, Greer KB, Yadlapati R, Spechler SJ. ACG Clinical Guideline for the Diagnosis and Management of Gastroesophageal Reflux Disease. Am J Gastroenterol. 2022;117(1):27-56.

odynophagia, persistent vomiting, or a strong family history of gastrointestinal cancer (**Box 1**).

Therefore, evaluation in the primary care setting may also include checking a hematogram and weight trend. The purpose of endoscopic evaluation in this setting is to assess for alternate mucosal etiologies (such as malignancy, eosinophilic esophagitis, pill esophagitis, infectious esophagitis) but also manifestations or complications of GERD (such as reflux-mediated strictures, reflux esophagitis, or BE).

Management

Management of GERD symptoms in the primary care setting features a multimodal approach comprised of lifestyle modifications and/or pharmacologic therapy.

Lifestyle modifications

Lifestyle modifications should be considered for all patients with GERD symptoms, and represent useful complements to pharmacologic therapy (**Table 1**). Randomized data have demonstrated improvements in nocturnal GERD symptoms and esophageal acid exposure with specific sleep positioning, specifically head of bed elevation and lying left-side down (left lateral decubitus), which position the esophagus and stomach more optimally.[12–15] In practice, these interventions can be facilitated with wedges, dedicated reflux pillows, and/or bricks or books to elevate the head of bed.

In addition to these sleep modifications, dietary modifications can provide benefits for GERD symptoms. Prolonging the dinner-to-bed interval, particularly by the avoidance of meals within 2 to 3 hours of bedtime, can be helpful for nocturnal symptoms,[15] as short intervals between eating and bedtime are associated with increased GERD symptoms.[16,17] Esophageal symptom burden in obese individuals correlates with increased esophageal acid burden.[18] Weight gain may be associated with increased risks of GERD complications, and weight loss among overweight individuals can effectively reduce GERD symptoms as well as esophageal acid exposure.[19–22] Although patients often report specific dietary triggers for GERD symptoms, supporting data for the avoidance of specific foods or adoption of restrictive diets are limited.[23]

Although there is mixed evidence on tobacco cessation and GERD, prospective cohort data showed an association between smoking cessation and improvement in GERD symptoms for patients of normal body mass index.[24] In conjunction with the myriad benefits of tobacco cessation on health beyond GERD, this may reasonably be encouraged in patients with GERD. Although alcohol consumption may exacerbate GERD symptoms, there is limited evidence suggesting that alcohol cessation

Table 1		
Lifestyle modifications to be considered for gastroesophageal reflux disease symptoms		
Dietary	**Nocturnal**	**Other Modifications**
Weight loss in overweight or obese patients	Head of bed elevation	Diaphragmatic breathing
Avoidance of late evening meals (within 2–3 h of bedtime)	Left lateral decubitus sleeping position	Tobacco cessation
Elimination of dietary symptom triggers		

Adapted from Katz PO, Dunbar KB, Schnoll-Sussman FH, Greer KB, Yadlapati R, Spechler SJ. ACG Clinical Guideline for the Diagnosis and Management of Gastroesophageal Reflux Disease. Am J Gastroenterol. 2022;117(1):27-56.

reduces esophageal acid exposure.[25] A recent randomized controlled trial demonstrated that diaphragmatic breathing exercises are associated with reduced numbers of postprandial reflux events, and may represent a practical and safe intervention for GERD symptoms.[26]

Pharmacotherapy

Antacids and H2 receptor antagonists. Readily available antacid formulations neutralize stomach acidity and are often utilized by patients for rapid, on-demand control of typical reflux symptoms (**Box 2**),[27,28] but their utility for long-term use or healing of erosive esophagitis is limited.[29] Alginate preparations may also be effective for symptomatic relief of GERD, though not as effective as PPI therapy.[30]

Antacids and H2 receptor antagonists (H2RA) medications, also known as H2-blockers, reduce gastric acid secretion by competing for and reversibly binding to H2 receptors found on gastric parietal cells. Although H2RAs are less effective than PPIs for acid-peptic indications,[31] H2RAs have shown some efficacy for the healing of erosive esophagitis.[32] H2RAs can play a role in milder GERD symptoms and/or on-demand dosing, as well as for step-down treatment after successful PPI trials.[33] Although data suggest some improvements in the control of nocturnal acid breakthrough in patients with the addition of bedtime H2RA to PPI taken twice daily, this benefit is quickly lost in the setting of tachyphylaxis (tolerance), and there are no significant differences in intragastric acid control with or without the addition of H2RA in patients on PPI after approximately 1 month of treatment.[34,35]

Proton pump inhibitor therapy. PPI formulations represent the most widely prescribed and evidence-based pharmacologic therapies for GERD in US clinical practice at present. PPI formulations suppress gastric acid secretion by irreversibly binding to and inhibiting the hydrogen-potassium ATPase pump found on the luminal surface of gastric parietal cells.[28] For patients presenting with typical GERD symptoms of heartburn and/or regurgitation without alarm features, society guidance recommends initiating a trial of empiric PPI therapy, typically once daily taken 30 to 60 minutes before breakfast, for 8 weeks.[3] Regarding the choice of PPI, a prior investigation has demonstrated general equivalence between PPI formulations for symptom relief or healing of erosive esophagitis.[36]

This initial management strategy can serve both diagnostic and therapeutic purposes.[28] Meta-analysis has demonstrated that 72% of patients with erosive esophagitis attain complete relief of heartburn after 4 weeks of PPI therapy.[37] PPI trials do have limitations; a meta-analysis demonstrated that the pooled sensitivity of a PPI trial

---

Box 2
Classes of pharmacologic therapy for gastroesophageal reflux disease

Pharmacologic Treatment Options for GERD
- On-demand antacids
- H2 receptor antagonists (H2RAs)
- Proton pump inhibitors (PPIs)
- Potassium-competitive acid blockers (PCABs)
- Potential adjunctive therapies (alginates, baclofen, prokinetics)

Data from Patel A, Yadlapati R. Diagnosis and Management of Refractory Gastroesophageal Reflux Disease. Gastroenterol Hepatol (N Y). 2021;17(7):305-315.

---

in resolving heartburn was 78% with abnormal endoscopy and ambulatory pH monitoring as the gold standard, but specificity was only 54%.[38,39]

For patients without an adequate symptom response with once-daily PPI therapy, the dose may be increased to twice daily; however, in the setting of persistent symptoms, referral to gastroenterology for further evaluation is appropriate.[28,40,41] Twice-daily dosing of even the relatively least potent PPI (pantoprazole at 20 mg) is at least equal if not superior to once-daily higher dosing of the most potent PPIs (such as rabeprazole at 40 mg).[42,43] There is no proven benefit to increasing beyond twice-daily dosing.[28]

For patients who obtain adequate symptom response with PPI therapy, expert guidance recommends tapering to the lowest effective dose for symptom control.[41] This may include conversion of dosing to on-demand therapy for symptoms, as well as consideration of H2RA for step-down therapy. For patients who require chronic PPI therapy for typical GERD symptoms beyond 1 year, referral to gastroenterology may be considered for ambulatory reflux monitoring to help guide the appropriateness of lifelong pharmacologic therapy.[41] Gastroenterology evaluation may provide additional diagnostic information to support PPI continuation or discontinuation, identify contributing co-morbid pathology, or facilitate discussion of non-PPI management options.

Although there have been concerns raised about the potential adverse effects of long-term PPI use, these have stemmed primarily from associations based on observational data.[44,45] The findings of these typically weak associations, which do not establish cause-and-effect relationships, are subject to confounding by indication (where the indication for which the PPI was prescribed is associated with the purported effect), protopathic bias (where the PPI was prescribed in response to early symptoms of an undiagnosed condition), and other biases.[3,46] The highest-quality data available on PPI safety to date are a large randomized controlled trial in which nearly 18,000 adults on rivaroxaban, aspirin, or both were randomized to pantoprazole 40 mg daily or placebo, and followed at 6-month intervals for a median duration of 3 years.[47] This study found no significant differences between the PPI and placebo groups in terms of pneumonia, fractures, chronic kidney disease, diabetes, chronic obstructive lung disease, dementia, cardiovascular disease, cancer, hospitalizations, or all-cause mortality. Only enteric infections were slightly more common in the PPI group (1.4% vs 1.0%). Further, propensity-score weighting analysis of retrospective data of United States veterans who tested positive for coronavirus disease-19 (COVID-19) showed similar rates of severe COVID composite outcomes between PPI users and PPI non-users, providing further reassurance around PPI safety in the COVID era.[48]

Despite the data supporting the safety of PPI medications, clinicians should still be vigilant to taper PPI therapy to the lowest effective dose for symptoms, and deprescribe if appropriate, in the absence of an indication for chronic PPI use. Those patients with severe reflux esophagitis, reflux-mediated stenosis, BE, eosinophilic esophagitis, idiopathic pulmonary fibrosis, and/or at high risk for upper gastrointestinal bleeding should generally not be considered for PPI discontinuation and/or deprescribing.[49] Overall, however, in the appropriate clinical settings, the proven benefits of PPI therapy outweigh any theoretical risks.[3]

Potassium-competitive acid blockers. Potassium-competitive acid blockers (PCABs) are gaining expanded approval for their utility in acid-peptic diseases.[50] They can more rapidly increase intragastric pH when compared with PPIs, by inhibition of proton pump potassium-exchange channels. In contrast to PPI formulations, PCABs are acid stable, facilitate reversible inhibition, and may be dosed independent of mealtimes.[51,52] Based on their availability, they may represent a potential therapeutic option for GERD and other acid-peptic disorders.

When to Refer

In general, among patients with suspected GERD symptoms, primary care providers should consider referral to gastroenterology for patients who present with alarm features (see **Box 1**), those with symptoms refractory to appropriate PPI trials, those with extra-esophageal symptoms in the absence of apparent non-GERD etiologies, those meeting criteria for screening for BE, and/or those with concerns or questions about the appropriateness of long-term PPI maintenance therapy (see **Fig. 1**).[3] Gastroenterology specialist evaluation facilitates advanced diagnostic testing, such as upper endoscopy for direct visualization and/or biopsies of the esophagus, esophageal high-resolution manometry (HRM) to evaluate esophageal motor function, and/or ambulatory reflux monitoring (typically performed off PPI in the absence of confirmatory evidence for GERD), to better identify the underlying causes of patient symptoms and, in turn, determine appropriate management. If indeed Gastroenterology evaluation points toward refractory GERD generating persisting symptoms, individualized management[41] may include escalation of therapy via pharmacologic (including adjunctive medication options), endoscopic (ie, transoral incisionless fundoplication), or surgical (ie, fundoplication, magnetic sphincter augmentation,[53] gastric bypass) approaches.[1]

Importantly, patients who meet the criteria for screening for BE should be referred for Gastroenterology evaluation (**Box 3**). BE is a metaplastic process that increases the risk of developing esophageal adenocarcinoma.[54–56] At this time, upper endoscopy is the most frequently utilized screening test for BE, though alternate non-endoscopic modalities remain of interest, including a recently developed capsule sponge device that can be used in the clinic setting.[54] Surveillance interval recommendations for patients found to have BE are based primarily on the degree of dysplasia and length of the BE segment; endoscopic eradication approaches are available and efficacious for dysplastic BE.[54] Lifelong PPI therapy is typically recommended for patients diagnosed with BE. Of note, repeat screening is not typically recommended for patients who have had a negative initial screening examination by endoscopy.

Gastroenterologist Specialist Evaluation

Most patients who are referred to gastroenterology for evaluation of suspected GERD symptoms will undergo upper endoscopy as an initial diagnostic step.[2] In addition to ruling out alternate non-GERD mucosal etiologies for symptoms (such as eosinophilic,[57] pill, or infectious esophagitis, among others), endoscopy evaluates for evidence of GERD. Evidence for GERD on endoscopy includes severe reflux esophagitis (Los Angeles grades C or D), reflux-mediated stricture, or biopsy-proven BE.[1] Ideally, when the clinical setting allows, endoscopy can be performed

> **Box 3**
> **American College of Gastroenterology Guidelines for indications for Barrett's Esophagus screening**
>
> Indications for Screening for BE
>   Chronic GERD symptoms (weekly symptoms for at least 5 years)
>   *AND*
>   At least three additional risk factors for BE:
>   • Male sex
>   • Age >50 years
>   • White race
>   • Tobacco smoking
>   • Obesity
>   • First-degree relative with BE or esophageal adenocarcinoma
>
> *Data from* Shaheen NJ, Falk GW, Iyer PG, et al. Diagnosis and Management of Barrett's Esophagus: An Updated ACG Guideline. Am J Gastroenterol. 2022;117(4):559-587.

after PPI has been held for at least 2 to 4 weeks prior, to increase the diagnostic yield for GERD diagnosis and eosinophilic esophagitis.[3,58]

Per society guideline recommendations, after an unrevealing endoscopic exam, gastroenterology evaluation of suspected reflux symptoms may include esophageal function testing.[2] In this setting, esophageal HRM evaluates esophageal peristaltic function and serves to rule out esophageal motor disorders such as achalasia that can mimic GERD, to assess for behavioral disorders such as rumination or supragastric belching with post-prandial protocols, and to evaluate esophageal contractile reserve with multiple rapid swallow sequences to help tailor potential anti-reflux surgery.[59–61] Ambulatory reflux monitoring (which can be performed with trans nasal catheters or wireless probe modalities) serves to quantify reflux burden, calculate reflux-symptom association metrics, and phenotype patients to help guide appropriate management of patient symptoms.[5,62,63] In the absence of evidence for GERD on upper endoscopy as discussed above, ambulatory reflux monitoring is typically performed off PPI therapy (with PPI held for 5–7 days before testing).[2]

SUMMARY

Primary care providers frequently encounter suspected reflux symptoms in clinical practice. In the primary care setting, characterization of symptoms is paramount, as is evaluation for potential alarm symptoms or features. Although typical GERD symptoms of heartburn and/or regurgitation may deserve a PPI trial for symptom response, these alarm features should prompt gastroenterology referral for upper endoscopy. Patients with chest pain warrant prompt cardiac evaluation, and those with extra-esophageal symptoms, particularly if isolated without accompanying typical GERD symptoms, deserve appropriate work-up and/or specialist referral based on symptom presentation, which may include ENT, pulmonary, and/or allergy evaluation. Otherwise, if unrevealing, gastroenterology referral can facilitate upper endoscopic and/or esophageal function testing evaluation for accurate diagnosis, to guide individualized management tailored to patients and their symptoms.

CLINICS CARE POINTS

> • When seeing patients for suspected symptoms of GERD in the primary care setting, carefully evaluate for alarm symptoms that would prompt referral to gastroenterology for endoscopic evaluation.

- When seeing patients with typical reflux symptoms of heartburn and/or regurgitation in the absence of alarm features, a trial of PPI therapy may be prescribed with assessment of symptom response.
- When patients with typical reflux symptoms of heartburn and/or regurgitation obtain complete symptom relief with PPI trials, efforts should be made to wean PPI therapy to the lowest effective dosing for symptom control.
- When seeing patients for suspected reflux symptoms in the primary care setting, patients with risk factors for BE should be referred to Gastroenterology for consideration of screening.
- When seeing patients with chest pain in the primary care setting, cardiac evaluation is appropriate before consideration of gastrointestinal etiologies for symptoms.

DISCLOSURE

A. Patel: Service on the Editorial (Review) Board of *Gastroenterology*, consultant for Medpace and Renexxion. The contents of this article do not represent the views of the Department of Veterans Affairs or the United States Government. Other authors: none.

REFERENCES

1. Patel A, Yadlapati R. Diagnosis and Management of Refractory Gastroesophageal Reflux Disease. Gastroenterol Hepatol 2021;17:305–15.
2. Gyawali CP, Carlson DA, Chen JW, et al. ACG Clinical Guidelines: Clinical Use of Esophageal Physiologic Testing. Am J Gastroenterol 2020;115:1412–28.
3. Katz PO, Dunbar KB, Schnoll-Sussman FH, et al. ACG Clinical Guideline for the Diagnosis and Management of Gastroesophageal Reflux Disease. Am J Gastroenterol 2022;117:27–56.
4. Gyawali CP, Kahrilas PJ, Savarino E, et al. Modern diagnosis of GERD: the Lyon Consensus. Gut 2018;67:1351–62.
5. Patel A, Gyawali CP. Gastroesophageal Reflux Monitoring. J Am Med Assoc 2018;319:1271.
6. The global, regional, and national burden of gastro-oesophageal reflux disease in 195 countries and territories, 1990-2017: a systematic analysis for the Global Burden of Disease Study 2017. Lancet Gastroenterol Hepatol 2020;5:561–81.
7. El-Serag HB, Sweet S, Winchester CC, et al. Update on the epidemiology of gastro-oesophageal reflux disease: a systematic review. Gut 2014;63:871–80.
8. Peery AF, Crockett SD, Murphy CC, et al. Burden and Cost of Gastrointestinal, Liver, and Pancreatic Diseases in the United States: Update 2021. Gastroenterology 2022;162:621–44.
9. Vakil N, van Zanten SV, Kahrilas P, et al. The Montreal definition and classification of gastroesophageal reflux disease: a global evidence-based consensus. Am J Gastroenterol 2006;101:1900–20 [quiz: 1943].
10. Sharma P, Yadlapati R. Pathophysiology and treatment options for gastroesophageal reflux disease: looking beyond acid. Ann N Y Acad Sci 2021;1486:3–14.
11. Kushner PR. Role of the primary care provider in the diagnosis and management of heartburn. Curr Med Res Opin 2010;26:759–65.
12. Schuitenmaker JM, van Dijk M, Oude Nijhuis RAB, et al. Associations Between Sleep Position and Nocturnal Gastroesophageal Reflux: A Study Using

Concurrent Monitoring of Sleep Position and Esophageal pH and Impedance. Am J Gastroenterol 2022;117:346–51.

13. Khoury RM, Camacho-Lobato L, Katz PO, et al. Influence of spontaneous sleep positions on nighttime recumbent reflux in patients with gastroesophageal reflux disease. Am J Gastroenterol 1999;94:2069–73.

14. van Herwaarden MA, Katzka DA, Smout AJ, et al. Effect of different recumbent positions on postprandial gastroesophageal reflux in normal subjects. Am J Gastroenterol 2000;95:2731–6.

15. Schuitenmaker JM, Kuipers T, Smout A, et al. Systematic review: Clinical effectiveness of interventions for the treatment of nocturnal gastroesophageal reflux. Neurogastroenterol Motil 2022;e14385.

16. Piesman M, Hwang I, Maydonovitch C, et al. Nocturnal reflux episodes following the administration of a standardized meal. Does timing matter? Am J Gastroenterol 2007;102:2128–34.

17. Ness-Jensen E, Hveem K, El-Serag H, et al. Lifestyle Intervention in Gastroesophageal Reflux Disease. Clin Gastroenterol Hepatol 2016;14:175–82.e1-3.

18. Rogers BD, Patel A, Wang D, et al. Higher Esophageal Symptom Burden in Obese Subjects Results From Increased Esophageal Acid Exposure and Not From Dysmotility. Clin Gastroenterol Hepatol 2020;18:1719–26.

19. Singh M, Lee J, Gupta N, et al. Weight loss can lead to resolution of gastroesophageal reflux disease symptoms: a prospective intervention trial. Obesity (Silver Spring) 2013;21:284–90.

20. Ness-Jensen E, Lindam A, Lagergren J, et al. Weight loss and reduction in gastroesophageal reflux. A prospective population-based cohort study: the HUNT study. Am J Gastroenterol 2013;108:376–82.

21. Fraser-Moodie CA, Norton B, Gornall C, et al. Weight loss has an independent beneficial effect on symptoms of gastro-oesophageal reflux in patients who are overweight. Scand J Gastroenterol 1999;34:337–40.

22. Mathus-Vliegen LM, Tytgat GN. Twenty-four-hour pH measurements in morbid obesity: effects of massive overweight, weight loss and gastric distension. Eur J Gastroenterol Hepatol 1996;8:635–40.

23. Kaltenbach T, Crockett S, Gerson LB. Are lifestyle measures effective in patients with gastroesophageal reflux disease? An evidence-based approach. Arch Intern Med 2006;166:965–71.

24. Ness-Jensen E, Lindam A, Lagergren J, et al. Tobacco smoking cessation and improved gastroesophageal reflux: a prospective population-based cohort study: the HUNT study. Am J Gastroenterol 2014;109:171–7.

25. Grande L, Manterola C, Ros E, et al. Effects of red wine on 24-hour esophageal pH and pressures in healthy volunteers. Dig Dis Sci 1997;42:1189–93.

26. Halland M, Bharucha AE, Crowell MD, et al. Effects of Diaphragmatic Breathing on the Pathophysiology and Treatment of Upright Gastroesophageal Reflux: A Randomized Controlled Trial. Am J Gastroenterol 2021;116:86–94.

27. Rohof WO, Bennink RJ, Smout AJ, et al. An alginate-antacid formulation localizes to the acid pocket to reduce acid reflux in patients with gastroesophageal reflux disease. Clin Gastroenterol Hepatol 2013;11:1585–91 [quiz: e90].

28. Gyawali CP, Fass R. Management of Gastroesophageal Reflux Disease. Gastroenterology 2018;154:302–18.

29. Weberg R, Berstad A. Symptomatic effect of a low-dose antacid regimen in reflux oesophagitis. Scand J Gastroenterol 1989;24:401–6.

30. Leiman DA, Riff BP, Morgan S, et al. Alginate therapy is effective treatment for GERD symptoms: a systematic review and meta-analysis. Dis Esophagus 2017;30:1–9.
31. van Pinxteren B, Sigterman KE, Bonis P, et al. Short-term treatment with proton pump inhibitors, H2-receptor antagonists and prokinetics for gastro-oesophageal reflux disease-like symptoms and endoscopy negative reflux disease. Cochrane Database Syst Rev 2010;Cd002095.
32. Chiba N, De Gara CJ, Wilkinson JM, et al. Speed of healing and symptom relief in grade II to IV gastroesophageal reflux disease: a meta-analysis. Gastroenterology 1997;112:1798–810.
33. Inadomi JM, Jamal R, Murata GH, et al. Step-down management of gastroesophageal reflux disease. Gastroenterology 2001;121:1095–100.
34. Peghini PL, Katz PO, Bracy NA, et al. Nocturnal recovery of gastric acid secretion with twice-daily dosing of proton pump inhibitors. Am J Gastroenterol 1998;93:763–7.
35. Fackler WK, Ours TM, Vaezi MF, et al. Long-term effect of H2RA therapy on nocturnal gastric acid breakthrough. Gastroenterology 2002;122:625–32.
36. Gralnek IM, Dulai GS, Fennerty MB, et al. Esomeprazole versus other proton pump inhibitors in erosive esophagitis: a meta-analysis of randomized clinical trials. Clin Gastroenterol Hepatol 2006;4:1452–8.
37. Weijenborg PW, Cremonini F, Smout AJ, et al. PPI therapy is equally effective in well-defined non-erosive reflux disease and in reflux esophagitis: a meta-analysis. Neurogastroenterol Motil 2012;24:747–757, e350.
38. Numans ME, Lau J, de Wit NJ, et al. Short-term treatment with proton-pump inhibitors as a test for gastroesophageal reflux disease: a meta-analysis of diagnostic test characteristics. Ann Intern Med 2004;140:518–27.
39. Aanen MC, Weusten BL, Numans ME, et al. Effect of proton-pump inhibitor treatment on symptoms and quality of life in GERD patients depends on the symptom-reflux association. J Clin Gastroenterol 2008;42:441–7.
40. Roman S, Gyawali CP, Savarino E, et al. Ambulatory reflux monitoring for diagnosis of gastro-esophageal reflux disease: Update of the Porto consensus and recommendations from an international consensus group. Neurogastroenterol Motil 2017;29:1–15.
41. Yadlapati R, Gyawali CP, Pandolfino JE. AGA Clinical Practice Update on the Personalized Approach to the Evaluation and Management of GERD: Expert Review. Clin Gastroenterol Hepatol 2022;20:984–94.e1.
42. Graham DY, Tansel A. Interchangeable Use of Proton Pump Inhibitors Based on Relative Potency. Clin Gastroenterol Hepatol 2018;16:800–8.e7.
43. Fass R, Murthy U, Hayden CW, et al. Omeprazole 40 mg once a day is equally effective as lansoprazole 30 mg twice a day in symptom control of patients with gastro-oesophageal reflux disease (GERD) who are resistant to conventional-dose lansoprazole therapy-a prospective, randomized, multi-centre study. Aliment Pharmacol Ther 2000;14:1595–603.
44. Islam MM, Poly TN, Walther BA, et al. Adverse outcomes of long-term use of proton pump inhibitors: a systematic review and meta-analysis. Eur J Gastroenterol Hepatol 2018;30:1395–405.
45. Vaezi MF, Yang YX, Howden CW. Complications of Proton Pump Inhibitor Therapy. Gastroenterology 2017;153:35–48.
46. Rajan P, Iglay K, Rhodes T, et al. Risk of bias in non-randomized observational studies assessing the relationship between proton-pump inhibitors and adverse

kidney outcomes: a systematic review. Therap Adv Gastroenterol 2022;15. 17562848221074183.

47. Moayyedi P, Eikelboom JW, Bosch J, et al. Safety of Proton Pump Inhibitors Based on a Large, Multi-Year, Randomized Trial of Patients Receiving Rivaroxaban or Aspirin. Gastroenterology 2019;157:682–91.e2.

48. Shah S, Halvorson A, McBay B, et al. Proton-pump inhibitor use is not associated with severe COVID-19-related outcomes: a propensity score-weighted analysis of a national veteran cohort. Gut 2022;71:1447–50.

49. Targownik LE, Fisher DA, Saini SD. AGA Clinical Practice Update on De-Prescribing of Proton Pump Inhibitors: Expert Review. Gastroenterology 2022; 162:1334–42.

50. Wong N, Reddy A, Patel A. Potassium-Competitive Acid Blockers: Present and Potential Utility in the Armamentarium for Acid Peptic Disorders. Gastroenterol Hepatol 2022;18:693–700.

51. Abdel-Aziz Y, Metz DC, Howden CW. Review article: potassium-competitive acid blockers for the treatment of acid-related disorders. Aliment Pharmacol Ther 2021;53:794–809.

52. Oshima T, Miwa H. Potent Potassium-competitive Acid Blockers: A New Era for the Treatment of Acid-related Diseases. J Neurogastroenterol Motil 2018;24: 334–44.

53. Patel A, Gyawali CP. The role of magnetic sphincter augmentation (MSA) in the gastroesophageal reflux disease (GERD) treatment pathway: the gastroenterology perspective. Dis Esophagus 2023. https://doi.org/10.1093/dote/doad005. doad005.

54. Shaheen NJ, Falk GW, Iyer PG, et al. Diagnosis and Management of Barrett's Esophagus: An Updated ACG Guideline. Am J Gastroenterol 2022;117:559–87.

55. Qumseya BJ, Bukannan A, Gendy S, et al. Systematic review and meta-analysis of prevalence and risk factors for Barrett's esophagus. Gastrointest Endosc 2019; 90:707–17.e1.

56. Thrift AP. Global burden and epidemiology of Barrett oesophagus and oesophageal cancer. Nat Rev Gastroenterol Hepatol 2021;18:432–43.

57. Posner S, Boyd A, Patel A. Dysphagia in a 34-Year-Old Woman. JAMA 2020;3(7): 660–1.

58. Odiase E, Schwartz A, Souza RF, et al. New Eosinophilic Esophagitis Concepts Call for Change in Proton Pump Inhibitor Management Before Diagnostic Endoscopy. Gastroenterology 2018;154:1217–21.e3.

59. Patel A, Posner S, Gyawali CP. Esophageal High-Resolution Manometry in Gastroesophageal Reflux Disease. JAMA 2018;320:1279–80.

60. Garbarino S, Horton A, Patel A. The Utility of Esophageal Motility Testing in Gastroesophageal Reflux Disease (GERD). Curr Gastroenterol Rep 2019;21:37.

61. Horton A, Jawitz N, Patel A. The Clinical Utility of Provocative Maneuvers at Esophageal High-resolution Manometry (HRM). J Clin Gastroenterol 2021;55: 95–102.

62. Patel A, Sayuk GS, Gyawali CP. Parameters on esophageal pH-impedance monitoring that predict outcomes of patients with gastroesophageal reflux disease. Clin Gastroenterol Hepatol 2015;13:884–91.

63. Patel A, Sayuk GS, Kushnir VM, et al. GERD phenotypes from pH-impedance monitoring predict symptomatic outcomes on prospective evaluation. Neurogastroenterol Motil 2016;28:513–21.

Peptic Ulcer Disease

Emily Tuerk, MD*, Sara Doss, MD, Kevin Polsley, MD

KEYWORDS

- Peptic ulcer disease • Epigastric pain • H. pylori • NSAIDs • GI bleeding

KEY POINTS

- Most patients with PUD have a relapsing course with intermittent symptoms of gnawing or burning epigastric pain.
- The two biggest risk factors for peptic ulcer disease are H pylori infection and NSAID use, and primary care physicians should screen for these conditions.
- Dyspepsia guidelines recommend EGD for patients with PUD over age 60 and H. pylori testing for patients under age 60.
- H. pylori treatment should be guided by local resistance rates and patient specific factors.
- For patients with NSAID induced PUD, PPI therapy should be initiated and NSAID use discontinued if possible.

INTRODUCTION

Peptic ulcer disease is defined as a mucosal break in the stomach and small intestine that reaches the submucosa.[1] Erosions are small, superficial breaks while peptic ulcers generally are defined as 5 mm or larger.[2] For decades, it was believed that human emotional stress was the main factor in the development of the disease.[3] Treatments were often surgical and the condition for many people was lifelong. Now we know that peptic ulcer disease is most often related to *Helicobacter pylori* infection or NSAID use. Although the *H pylori* organism was discovered in the early 1980s, there was initial skepticism at its role in disease.[3] It was not until 1994 that the National Institutes of Health Consensus Development Conference on *H pylori* in Peptic Ulcer Disease came together to make recommendations regarding the treatment of *H pylori* with antibiotics and antisecretory medications.[4] This began a new era in the treatment of PUD.

Since that time, the prevalence of *H pylori* infection has been declining in the United States,[5] but the overall burden of disease remains significant. There are an estimated 230,000 cases of upper GI bleed presenting to the ER and over 75% of those patients require admission.[6] Complications of *H pylori* infection include GI bleeding, perforation, and gastric outlet obstruction.[1] This article reviews the prevalence of disease,

Loyola University Chicago Stritch School of Medicine, Primary Care, 2160 South First Avenue, Mulcahy 2525, Maywood, IL 60153, USA
* Corresponding author.
E-mail address: etuerk@lumc.edu

Prim Care Clin Office Pract 50 (2023) 351–362
https://doi.org/10.1016/j.pop.2023.03.003
0095-4543/23/© 2023 Elsevier Inc. All rights reserved.

risk factors for disease, pathophysiology, presentation, diagnosis, and management of peptic ulcer disease focusing on both H. Pylori and NSAID-related disease.

PREVALENCE/INCIDENCE/RISK FACTORS

The incidence of PUD is approximately 1 case per 1000 person-years worldwide in the general population.[7] For those infected with H pylori the incidence of PUD is 1% per year.[8]

The incidence and prevalence of PUD are higher in individuals with H pylori. H pylori infection is usually acquired in childhood.[9] H pylori is spread when in close quarters and by fecal-oral route. Risk factors for H pylori disease are well documented (**Fig. 1**).[10] They include.

- Lower socioeconomic risk factors
- Increasing number of siblings, and
- The presence of an infected parent with an infected mother being higher risk than father.[9]

Additionally, there are known to be more infections in men than women.[9]

Geography also plays a role in H. pylori infection and therefore the risk of PUD. In countries with a higher rate of H pylori, the incidence of PUD is greater.[8] The highest prevalence of H. Pylori infection is in Africa at 70% and the lowest is in Western Europe at 34%.[8] In North America, H pylori rates vary with socioeconomic status and race/ethnicity[9] with prevalence being lowest in non-Hispanic whites.[9] Overall, the incidence of H pylori infection both in the US and abroad is downward trending over time[9,11] due to the improvement of hygiene, antibiotic use, and the use of proton pump inhibitors.

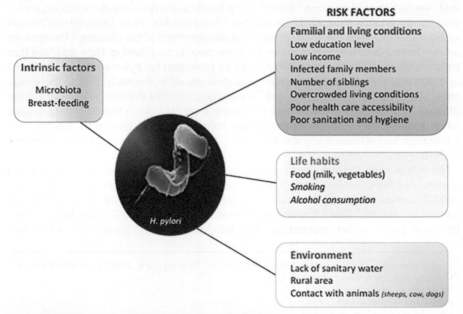

RISK FACTORS

Intrinsic factors
Microbiota
Breast-feeding

Familial and living conditions
Low education level
Low income
Infected family members
Number of siblings
Overcrowded living conditions
Poor health care accessibility
Poor sanitation and hygiene

Life habits
Food (milk, vegetables)
Smoking
Alcohol consumption

H. pylori

Environment
Lack of sanitary water
Rural area
Contact with animals (sheeps, cow, dogs)

Fig. 1. Risk factors associated to H. pylori infection. (*From* Kotilea K, Bontems P, Touati E. Epidemiology, Diagnosis and Risk Factors of Helicobacter pylori Infection. Adv Exp Med Biol. 2019;1149:17-33.)

NSAID use is also a major risk factor in the development of peptic ulcer disease.

Peptic ulcers are the most common cause of upper GI bleeding.[12] While mortality rates of hospitalized patients have decreased, there is still wide variability in fatality rates across the globe.[12] Peery and colleagues found in 1 year there were over 3700 deaths in the ER or while hospitalized related to upper GI bleeds.[4]

KEY POINTS

- The 2 biggest risk factors for PUD are *H pylori* infection and NSAID use.
- For patients infected with *H pylori* incidence of PUD is 1% per year
- Overall incidence of *H pylori* infection is downward trending over time.

Pathophysiology of Peptic Ulcer Disease

Peptic ulcers are caused by an imbalance between aggressive and defensive factors in the gastrointestinal mucosa.[13]

Gastric acid and the proteolytic enzyme pepsin were originally thought to be large contributors to the development of ulcers. This led to the consideration that decreasing acid production was key in the prevention and treatment of ulcers. It was not until after the discovery of *H pylori* (previously *Campylobacter pyloridis*) by Warren and Marshal in 1982 that led the rethinking of PUD.[14] It shifted from a disease solely of acid dysregulation to an infectious disease.[14]

Acid production in the stomach is key to mucosal defense and protein hydrolysis and digestion. After a meal, gastric acid is secreted. Gastric acid also causes the release of somatostatin from antral D cells, which acts as a negative feedback to inhibit further gastric acid secretion from G cells and parietal cells. Too much acid production can lead to gastric or duodenal mucosal erosion. Interestingly, high gastric acid levels are not commonly found in patients with gastric ulcers, and are even less common in those with duodenal ulcers.[13]

Mucosal defense mechanisms are also essential in protection against erosions and ultimately ulcerations. Mucosal defense mechanisms include bicarbonate secretion, adequate mucosal blood flow, and cell repair. These defense mechanisms are regulated by prostaglandins, nitric acid, and other proteins.[15]

H.pylori, a gram-negative spiral and flagellated urease-producing bacterium, has several mechanisms by which it can contribute to or cause ulcerations (**Fig. 2**). In patients with *H pylori*, there appears to be a decreased number of antral D cells, leading to less secretion of somatostatin.[14] Without the negative feedback of somatostatin there are ultimately higher levels of gastric acid. *H pylori* also has high urease activity leading to increased production of ammonia.[15] Ammonia protects the organism from highly acidic environment.[14] Local ammonia production changes the physiology of antral D cells and ultimately increases acid production. Ammonia itself can also contribute to cell damage.[15] *H pylori* also attaches itself to epithelial cells and causes a pro-inflammatory response locally. The bacteria synthesizes and releases proteases that damage mucosa and the host epithelial cells release cytokines IL-8, TNF-alpha, IL-6 that also cause local inflammation and damage.[15] Some *H pylori* isolates also produce toxins that are more pathogenic, leading to more cell damage. These isolates carry a cytotoxin-associated gene (cagA gene) which is a marker for more virulent strains.[13] Other markers of more virulent strains include the vacuolating cytotoxin and the blood group antigen-binding adhesion.[2]

NSAID and low-dose aspirin use have been identified as a major cause of gastric and duodenal ulcerations as well.[14] In fact, those patients with GI bleeds are often

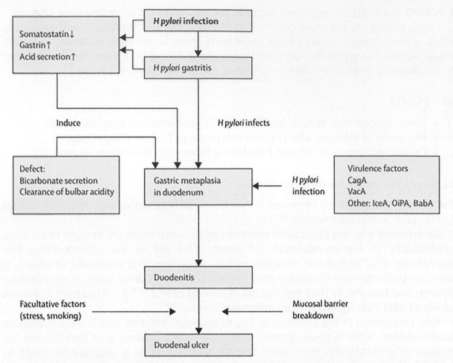

Fig. 2. Mechanisms by which H pylori cause or contribute to ulcerations. (*Reprinted with permission from* Elsevier. The Lancet, October 2009, 374 (9699), 1449-1461.)

associated with NSAID use. NSAID use has also been associated with spontaneous perforation.[14] NSAIDS do contribute to local mucosal erosion and injury.[15] NSAIDS also inhibit the production of prostaglandins, thereby lowering the mucosal defense mechanisms. Any NSAID can cause ulcer formation by this mechanism, even enteric-coated NSAIDS. Some individuals also have a genetic polymorphism of cytochrome P450 2C9 which can delay the metabolism of NSAIDS, increasing gastric mucosa exposure time to NSAIDS.[16]

Zollinger-Ellison syndrome (ZES) is a rare condition that accounts for a small proportion of gastroduodenal ulcers.[15] This condition is associated with massive secretion of gastrin (secondary to a gastrinoma) and acid production leading to multiple, recurrent ulcers. Gastrin levels are often over 1000 pg/mL. These ulcers can present in unusual locations, such as the distal duodenum or jejunum.

There are several host mechanisms and environmental factors that can alter the balance between protective defense mechanisms and aggressive factors. These include tobacco use, alcohol and drug use, and psychological stress. In fact, the incidence of PUD in smokers versus nonsmokers is almost twice as high.[17] However, none of these factors are proven etiologies of ulcer formation but can influence their formation.[14]

Other factors that can contribute to or cause ulceration include.

- Hypovolemia
- Critical illness leading to Cushing or Curling ulcers
- Malignancy (adenocarcinoma, lymphoma)
- Medications including bisphosphonates, corticosteroids, SSRIs, sirolimus.[18]

KEY POINTS

- Peptic ulcers are caused by an imbalance between aggressive and defensive factors in the gastrointestinal mucosa
- *H pylori* decreases somatostatin, increases ammonia through urease production, and produces local inflammation leading to ulcer formation. .
- Any NSAID, even enteric-coated NSAIDS, can cause local injury in the GI tract and lower GI defense.

CLINICAL PRESENTATION

Peptic ulcer disease has nonspecific symptoms but most classically is associated with epigastric pain usually described as gnawing or burning pain.[1] Primary care doctors should always screen patients with GI complaints about the use of NSAIDs and any history of known *H pylori* infection.[18] For most patients with PUD there is a relapsing course of illness and symptoms are intermittent.[18] Initial care may be sought in the primary care office setting.

Duodenal peptic ulcer disease is more likely to be associated with increased hunger and nocturnal abdominal pain.[1] These patients may feel symptom relief with eating.[14] On average these patients are younger ranging from 30 to 55 year old.[2] Ulcers are likely in the duodenal bulb or pyloric channel.[2]

Gastric peptic ulcer disease causes more postprandial pain, nausea, vomiting, and weight loss.[1] Gastric ulcers occur in older patients peaking in the 6th decade of life.[2] Ulcers are most likely to occur in the antrum and lesser curvature.[2]

Duodenal Peptic Ulcer Disease	Gastric Peptic Ulcer Disease
• Nocturnal abdominal pain	• Nausea, vomiting, weight loss
• Increased hunger	• Typically older patients ranging in 60s
• Typically younger patients - ranging 30–55yo	• Occur in the antrum and lesser curvature of the stomach
• Occur in duodenal bulb or pyloric channel	• Postprandial abdominal pain

Some patients at presentation may have both gastric and duodenal disease. Lee and colleagues found that approximately 10% of patients with PUD had disease in both the duodenum and the stomach.[19]

Patients with ulcers may not present with any abdominal pain and ulcers may be found because of evaluation for iron deficiency anemia. Lu and colleagues found that up to two-thirds of patients with peptic ulcer disease are asymptomatic.[20] There is some data that suggests patients with PUD caused by NSAIDS are more likely to have symptomatic disease[19] however PUD from any etiology can be asymptomatic. Some patients with ulcers found both in the stomach and the duodenum was asymptomatic.[19]

Patients may also present with complications of PUD at the time of their diagnosis. Bleeding is a frequent and often severe complication with highest risk in those over age 60.[14] Iron deficiency anemia may be an early warning sign of bleeding before a more severe event occurs. Significant bleeding can occur with no warning in nearly half of patients.[1] A brisk upper GI bleed may present with hematemesis, coffee ground emesis, or bright red blood per rectum. Bleeding from PUD may also present with melena. Other complications include perforation which has mortality rates reported up to 20%.[1] These patients may present with intense pain in the upper abdomen and back. While not common, persistent vomiting may be a sign of a gastric outlet obstruction and has a higher risk for associated gastrointestinal malignancy.[1]

PHYSICAL EXAMINATION

The physical examination is often normal though may show epigastric tenderness. All patients reporting frank melena or black stools should undergo a rectal examination to check for active bleeding. Tachycardia and orthostatic blood pressure may be found with upper GI bleed. Abdominal rigidity and rebound tenderness may be seen with perforation and subsequent peritonitis.

KEY POINTS

- Most patients with symptomatic PUD have a relapsing course of illness with intermittent symptoms including gnawing or burning epigastric pain. Primary care doctors should screen for NSAID use and history of *H pylori* infection.
- Pain from duodenal ulcers may improve with eating while gastric ulcers cause postprandial abdominal pain.
- A large proportion of patients with PUD can be asymptomatic.

Diagnosis

Endoscopy is required to establish the diagnosis of peptic ulcer disease.[1]

Outpatients with Epigastric Pain

Patients with predominant symptoms of epigastric pain for greater than 1 month in the outpatient setting should be stratified according to the dyspepsia guidelines.[21] Patients over 60 years of age will be referred to upper endoscopy and patients under 60 years of age will be tested for *H pylori* and treated if positive (**Fig. 3**).[21] Other patients with increased risk of gastrointestinal malignancies including those born in

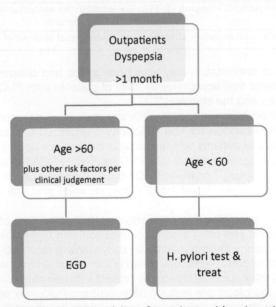

Fig. 3. Diagnostic protocol per ACG guidelines for patients with epigastric pain > 1m. (*Data from* Chey WD, Leontiadis GI, Howden CW, Moss SF. ACG Clinical Guideline: Treatment of Helicobacter pylori Infection [published correction appears in Am J Gastroenterol. 2018 Jul;113(7):1102]. Am J Gastroenterol. 2017;112(2):212-239.)

high-risk geographic areas or those with a family history of stomach cancer may also be screened with EGD according to clinical judgment.[21]

Imaging

Because patients present with acute presentations of abdominal pain and are often first seen in the ER, CT imaging may be done as part of initial work up. There are direct and indirect findings of uncomplicated PUD that may be detected on CT scan including submucosal edema, bowel wall thickening, adjacent fat stranding, and focal outpouching of the bowel lining.[22] These findings may help determine which patients in the ER need urgent GI consult and EGD.[22]

The Diagnosis of H pylori

When endoscopy confirms the diagnosis of peptic ulcer disease, biopsy of the mucosa in the antrum and body of the stomach is performed to test for *H pylori*.[14] The gold standard for *H pylori* diagnosis is done with histology. The rapid urease test has largely been replaced in the US with histology. The culture of the *H pylori* organism is difficult and expensive therefore culture of the organism is reserved for patients who have failed multiple treatment regimens and is done with sensitivity testing.[2] .

For patients not undergoing endoscopy, testing should be done with urea breath testing or stool antigen testing.[18] Both recent antibiotics and the use of PPIs can increase false negatives on breath testing.[2] If possible, PPIs should be held for 2 weeks and bismuth-containing medication and antibiotics should be held for 4 weeks before testing. Serology testing is the least preferred method.[18]

Patients Presenting with Upper Gastrointestinal Bleeding

For patients presenting to the ER with upper GI bleeding, the ACG Guidelines regarding Upper GI bleeding[23] dictate the timing of the examination. The use of the Glasgow-Blatchford scale has been shown to help risk stratify low-risk patients.[24] Low-risk patients with a Glasgow-Blatchford score equal to 0 or 1 (**Table 1**) may be discharged from the ER with close outpatient follow-up.[23] For other patients admitted with upper GI bleed, endoscopy should be performed within 24 hours.[23] Urgent GI consult is required to assist in completing EGD. In addition, all of these patients should be made NPO and started on intravenous PPI therapy. While awaiting definitive treatment, they require frequent monitoring of vital signs and serial laboratories from hemoglobin & hematocrit.

KEY POINTS

- Dyspepsia guidelines recommend EGD for patients over age 60 and *H. pylori* testing for patients under age 60.
- After EGD, *H. pylori* is diagnosed on biopsy with histology or rapid urease test.
- For patients not undergoing endoscopy, testing can be done with urea breath test or stool antigen testing. PPI should be held for 2 weeks before testing if possible. Antibiotics and bismuth-containing medications should be held for 4 weeks.
- For patients with upper GI bleed, Glasgow-Blatchford scale dictates the timing of GI consultation and endoscopy.

Management

Treatment of peptic ulcer disease is dependent on the primary cause and may include the eradication of *H. pylori*, avoidance of NSAID medications, and management of bleeding, if present. Prevention of ulcer recurrence is key to preventing future morbidity.

Table 1
Admission risk markers and associated score component values

Admission Risk Marker	Score Component Value
Blood urea (mmol/L)	
$\geq 6 \cdot 5 < 8 \cdot 0$	2
$\geq 8 \cdot 0 < 10 \cdot 0$	3
$\geq 10 \cdot 0 < 25 \cdot 0$	4
≥ 25	6
Hemoglobin (g/L) for men	
$\geq 120 < 130$	1
$\geq 100 < 120$	3
$< 10 \cdot 0$	6
Hemoglobin (g/L) for women	
$\geq 100 < 120$	1
< 100	6
Systollc blood pressure (mm Hg)	
100–109	1
90–99	2
< 90	3
Other markers	
Pulse ≥ 100 (per min)	1
Presentation with melaena	1
Presentation with syncope	2
Hepatic disease	2
Cardiac failure	2

Reprinted with permission from Elsevier. The Lancet, October 2000, 356 (9238), 1318-1321.

H. pylori-associated peptic ulcer disease:

Successful identification is important for the treatment of *H. pylori*-associated peptic ulcer disease. Successful treatment of *H. pylori* can lead to long-term resolution of peptic disease. Current ACG/CAG guidelines support a "test and treat" strategy for *H. pylori* for all patients under 60 years of age with dyspepsia using a noninvasive test such as stool antigen testing or breath testing.[21] In the past, standard treatment has included twice daily proton pump inhibitor (PPI) therapy and 2 antibiotics, Clarithromycin plus Amoxicillin or Metronidazole for 7 to 14 days (**Table 2**). However, increasing resistance to Clarithromycin has made eradication more challenging. If isolate susceptibility testing is available or local resistance rates are known, this can be used to guide therapy. ACG supports using local resistance rates greater than 15% as the cut off for using quadruple therapy (see **Table 2**).[9] New data from 2022 suggests that clarithromycin resistance rates in all US subregions and several European countries is over 15%.[25] Therefore, a bismuth-containing quadruple therapy or concomitant therapy (nonbismuth quadruple therapy) likely has greater eradication rates throughout the US.

Penicillin allergic patients should be treated with either Bismuth quadruple therapy or Clarithromycin triple therapy with Metronidazole. Patients with recent macrolide antibiotic exposure should be treated with either Bismuth quadruple therapy or for Levofloxacin triple therapy. Eradication testing should be performed in all patients 4 weeks after treatment, and PPI treatment should be withheld for at least 2 weeks

Table 2
Contrasting clarithromycin triple therapy vs. Bismuth quadruple therapy vs. concomitant (non-bismuth based quadruple therapy) vs. Levofloxacin triple therapy

Clarithromycin Triple Therapy 14 d	• PPI standard or double dose BID • Clarithromycin 500 mg BID • Amoxicillin 1 g BID or Metronidazole 500 mg TID
Bismuth Quadruple Therapy 10–14 d	• PPI standard dose BID • Tetracycline 500 mg QID • Metronidazole 250 mg QID or 500 mg TID/QID • Bismuth subcitrate 120–300 mg QID (or Bismuth subsalicylate 300 mg QID)
Levofloxacin Triple Therapy 10-14 days	• PPI standard dose BID • Levofloxacin 500 mg QD • Amoxicillin 1g BID
Concomitant Therapy 10-14 days	• PPI standard dose BID • Clarithromycin 500 mg BID • Amoxicillin 1 g BID • Metronidazole or Tinidazole 500 mg BID

Abbreviations: BID, twice daily; PPI, proton pump inhibitor, (assumes standard dosing); QD, once daily; QID, four times daily; TID, three times daily.

Data from Chey WD, Leontiadis GI, Howden CW, Moss SF. ACG Clinical Guideline: Treatment of Helicobacter pylori Infection [published correction appears in Am J Gastroenterol. 2018 Jul;113(7):1102]. *Am J Gastroenterol.* 2017;112(2):212-239.

before test of cure.[9] Patients should be warned about possible side effects of Metronidazole including metallic taste and GI upset.

Vonoprazan is an emerging therapy that is being used in place of traditional PPI therapy for the treatment of *H. pylori* infection. It was FDA approved in 2022 In combination with Amoxicillin alone or in combination with Clarithromycin for *H. pylori* treatment. It belongs to a class of drugs known as potassium-competitive acid blockers (P-CABs). Vonoprazan is stable in an acid environment, requires no acid activation, and has a longer half life than PPIs.[26] It has been shown to be more potent than traditional PPIs. Vonoprazan-Amoxicillin dual therapy has been shown to result in a 80% cure rate for *H. pylori* infection.[27]

Non-Steroidal Anti-Inflammatory Drug Associated Peptic Ulcer Disease

Discontinuation of the offending medication is important. PPI treatment is the mainstay of therapy for peptic ulcer disease. Treatment for 6 to 8 weeks achieves resolution in the vast majority of NSAID-induced PUD.[1] If the NSAID cannot be discontinued, resolution is slower.[14] Taking the NSAID with food may provide a buffer to decrease the risk of mucosal injury. Prevention of PUD for patients who must take chronic NSAID can include treatment with PPI, H2 receptor antagonist or misoprostol. COX-2 selective NSAIDs may also be used to lower the risk of developing PUD for patients who require NSAID therapy.[1] H2 receptor antagonists are not as effective in treatment and do not reduce the risk of gastric ulcer development.[1]

Duration of treatment with PPI therapy is dependent on a variety of factors including the severity of the underlying disease and complications. Chronic PPI therapy is not without significant potential side effects which can include increased risk of C difficile infection, decreased absorption of nutrients including calcium and magnesium, and gastric achlorhydria.[18] Malabsorption of nutrients can lead to increased bone fracture risk. PPI use has also been linked to renal complications including acute interstitial nephritis and increased incidence of chronic kidney disease.[28] Routine monitoring of GFR may be necessary, especially in the elderly or patients with CKD.

H. pylori Negative, NSAID Negative Peptic Ulcer Disease

The mainstay of management is again PPI therapy. If initial *H. pylori* testing is negative, PPI therapy should be started and the patient should be monitored for response. If the response is inadequate, other possible treatments can include prokinetic therapy, tricyclic antidepressant therapy or psychotherapy.[21] The risk of recurrence is higher in patients with idiopathic PUD.

Treatment Failures

Cases of treatment failure should prompt a careful history and evaluation of medication adherence. A twice daily PPI regimen may be prescribed with the first dose taken 30 minutes before breakfast, although evidence to support this is lacking.[1] *H. pylori* diagnostic testing is recommended if not performed initially. Other causes of persistent PUD should be considered including malignancy, atypical infections, and Zollinger-Ellison syndrome. Repeat EGD with biopsy of the ulcer edge to rule out malignancy should be considered.

Management of Peptic Ulcer Bleeding

Inpatient management of peptic ulcer bleeding is beyond the scope of this article. Prompt upper endoscopy is required for diagnosis and management. Following hospital discharge PPI therapy should be continued twice daily for 2 to 12 weeks depending on the size and features of the ulcer, followed by once daily therapy.[12] Following discharge the patient should have prompt follow-up with primary care and/or gastroenterology to evaluate for symptoms of bleeding and monitor hemoglobin levels.

When to Refer

Expert consultation should be sought for patients with resistant *H. pylori* infection, recurrent symptoms despite PPI treatment and *H. pylori* eradication, or history of severe peptic ulcer bleeding.

KEY POINTS

- *H. pylori* treatment should be guided by local resistance rates and patient-specific factors such as allergies and prior use of macrolide antibiotics
- Test of cure should be obtained for all patients treated for *H. pylori*
- For patients with NSAID-induced peptic disease, PPI therapy should be initiated and NSAIDs discontinued if possible
- If symptoms are not successfully treated with PPI use, prokinetic therapy, tricyclic antidepressant therapy or psychotherapy may be used and alternative diagnoses should be considered with a GI consultant.

Summary

Peptic ulcer disease is a common cause of dyspepsia. The two biggest risk factors for PUD are H. pylori infection and NSAID use. Diagnosis of PUD includes EGD for patients over age 60 and H. pylori testing for patients under age 60. Management of PUD includes the discontinuation of NSAIDS and treatment of H.pylori if applicable, driven by local susceptibility data.

CLINICS CARE POINTS

- Primary care physicians should screen patients with epigastric pain for NSAID use and assess for *H pylori* risk factors.

- EGD is needed to diagnose peptic ulcer disease. *H pylori* can be diagnosed during endoscopy via biopsy with histology or rapid urease test. If patients are not undergoing EGD, they can be tested with urea breath test or stool antigen. Antibiotics and proton pump inhibitors need to be held for at least 2 weeks before testing for *H pylori*. All patients positive for *H pylori* should be treated. After treatment, eradication testing should be performed in all patients 4 weeks after treatment and PPI therapy should be held for 2 weeks before test for cure.

- Given the high clarithromycin resistance rates in the US, bismuth-containing quadruple therapy or concomitant therapy (non-bismuth quadruple therapy) have greater eradication rates in the US.

DISCLOSURE

The authors have nothing to disclose.

ACKNOWLEDGMENTS

The authors would like to acknowledge Brian Liem, DO, Assistant Professor, Loyola University Chicago Stritch School of Medicine, Department of Gastroenterology, Maywood, IL, for his contributions to the paper.

REFERENCES

1. Lanas A, Chan FKL. Peptic ulcer disease. Lancet 2017;390(10094):613–24.
2. Lew E. Peptic Ulcer Disease. In: Greenberger NJ, Blumberg RS, Burakoff R. eds CURRENT Diagnosis & Treatment: Gastroenterology, Hepatology, & Endoscopy, 3e. McGraw Hill; 2016. Available at: https://accessmedicine-mhmedical-com. archer.luhs.org/content.aspx?bookid=1621&sectionid=105183277. Accessed October 07,2022.
3. Abbasi J, Marshall B. H. pylori 35 Years Later. JAMA 2017;317(14):1400–2.
4. Yamada T, Searle JG, Ahnen D, et al. Helicobacter pylori in Peptic Ulcer Disease. JAMA 1994;272(1):65–9.
5. Hooi JKY, Lai WY, Ng WK, et al. Global Prevalence of Helicobacter pylori Infection: Systematic Review and Meta-Analysis. Gastroenterology 2017;153(2): 420–9.
6. Peery AF, Crockett SD, Murphy CC, et al. Burden and Cost of Gastrointestinal, Liver, and Pancreatic Diseases in the United States: Update 2018. Gastroenterology 2019;156(1):254–72.e11 [published correction appears in Gastroenterology. 2019 May;156(6):1936].
7. Lin KJ, García Rodríguez LA, Hernández-Diaz S. Systematic review of peptic ulcer disease incidence rates: do studies without validation provide reliable estimates? Pharmacoepidemiol Drug Saf 2011;20(7):718–28.
8. Kuipers EJ, Thijs JC, Festen HP. The prevalence of Helicobacter pylori in peptic ulcer disease. Aliment Pharmacol Ther 1995;9(Suppl 2):59–69.
9. Chey WD, Leontiadis GI, Howden CW, et al. ACG Clinical Guideline: Treatment of Helicobacter pylori Infection. Am J Gastroenterol 2017;112(2):212–39 [published correction appears in Am J Gastroenterol. 2018 Jul;113(7):1102].

10. Kotilea K, Bontems P, Touati E. Epidemiology, Diagnosis and Risk Factors of Helicobacter pylori Infection. Adv Exp Med Biol 2019;1149:17–33.
11. Azhari H, King JA, Coward S, et al. The Global Incidence of Peptic Ulcer Disease Is Decreasing Since the Turn of the 21st Century: A Study of the Organisation for Economic Co-Operation and Development (OECD). Am J Gastroenterol 2022; 117(9):1419–27.
12. Laine L. CLINICAL PRACTICE. Upper Gastrointestinal Bleeding Due to a Peptic Ulcer. N Engl J Med 2016;374(24):2367–76.
13. Andreoli TE, Carpenter GL. Cecil Essentials of Medicine. 2004, pgs 351–7.
14. Malfertheiner P, Chan FK, McColl KE. Peptic ulcer disease. Lancet 2009; 374(9699):1449–61.
15. Del Valle J. Chapter 324: Peptic Ulcer Disease and Related Disorders.In: Loscalzo J, Fauci A, Kasper D, Hauser S, Longo D, Jameson J. eds Harrison's Principles of Internal Medicine, 21e. McGraw Hill; 2022. Accessed October 07, 2022. Available at: https://accessmedicine-mhmedical-com.archer.luhs.org/content.aspx?bookid=3095&sectionid=259856983
16. Pilotto A, Seripa D, Franceschi M, et al. Genetic susceptibility to nonsteroidal anti-inflammatory drug-related gastroduodenal bleeding: role of cytochrome P450 2C9 polymorphisms. Gastroenterology 2007;133(2):465–71.
17. Garrow D, Delegge MH. Risk factors for gastrointestinal ulcer disease in the US population. Dig Dis Sci 2010;55(1):66–72.
18. Kavitt RT, Lipowska AM, Anyane-Yeboa A, et al. Diagnosis and Treatment of Peptic Ulcer Disease. Am J Med 2019;132(4):447–56.
19. Lee SP, Sung IK, Kim JH, et al. Risk Factors for the Presence of Symptoms in Peptic Ulcer Disease. Clin Endosc 2017;50(6):578–84.
20. Lu CL, Chang SS, Wang SS, et al. Silent peptic ulcer disease: frequency, factors leading to "silence," and implications regarding the pathogenesis of visceral symptoms. Gastrointest Endosc 2004;60(1):34–8.
21. Moayyedi P, Lacy BE, Andrews CN, et al. ACG and CAG Clinical Guideline: Management of Dyspepsia. Am J Gastroenterol 2017;112(7):988–1013 [published correction appears in Am J Gastroenterol. 2017 Sep;112(9):1484].
22. Baghdanian AH, Baghdanian AA, Puppala S, et al. Imaging Manifestations of Peptic Ulcer Disease on Computed Tomography. Semin Ultrasound CT MR 2018;39(2):183–92.
23. Laine L, Barkun AN, Saltzman JR, et al. ACG Clinical Guideline: Upper Gastrointestinal and Ulcer Bleeding [published correction appears in Am J Gastroenterol. 2021 Nov 1;116(11):2309]. Am J Gastroenterol 2021;116(5):899–917.
24. Blatchford O, Murray WR, Blatchford M. A risk score to predict need for treatment for upper-gastrointestinal haemorrhage. Lancet 2000;356(9238):1318–21.
25. Mégraud F, Graham DY, Howden CW, et al. Rates of Antimicrobial Resistance in Helicobacter pylori Isolates from Clinical Trial Patients Across the US and Europe [published online ahead of print, 2022 Sep 30]. Am J Gastroenterol 2022. https://doi.org/10.14309/ajg.0000000000002045.
26. Miftahussurur M, Pratama Putra B, Yamaoka Y. The Potential Benefits of Vonoprazan as Helicobacter pylori Infection Therapy. Pharmaceuticals (Basel) 2020; 13(10):276.
27. Graham DY, Dore MP. Update on the Use of Vonoprazan: A Competitive Acid Blocker. Gastroenterology 2018;154(3):462–6.
28. Freedberg DE, Kim LS, Yang YX. The Risks and Benefits of Long-term Use of Proton Pump Inhibitors: Expert Review and Best Practice Advice From the American Gastroenterological Association. Gastroenterology 2017;152(4):706–15.

Approach to Elevated Liver Enzymes

Jessica Rosenberg, MD, MHS[a],*, Orlando Sola, MD, MPH[b], Adam Visconti, MD, MPH[c]

KEYWORDS

- Transaminitis • Liver function tests • Non-alcoholic fatty liver • NAFLD
- Alcohol-associated liver disease • Hepatitis • Drug-induced liver injury • DILI

KEY POINTS

- Abnormalities in liver enzymes are most associated with non-alcoholic fatty liver disease, and alcoholic liver disease, as well as common infectious diseases such hepatitis B and C.
- The R ratio can be used to determine the type of liver injury pattern, and to guide subsequent work-up of abnormal liver testing.
- The primary care physician plays a crucial role in preventing and diagnosing drug-induced liver injury.
- Hepatitis C can successfully be diagnosed and treated in the primary care setting.

INTRODUCTION

Abnormal liver tests are one of the most common challenges in the primary care setting. The standard liver tests (often referred to as "liver function tests [LFTs]") typically include alanine transaminase (ALT) and aspartate transaminase (AST), alkaline phosphatase (ALP), gamma-glutamyl transferase (GGT), serum bilirubin, prothrombin time (PT), the international normalized ratio (INR), and albumin.

Evaluation should be guided by both the clinical presentation and the pattern of injury.

In this article, we will focus mainly on the most common causes of abnormal liver testing, which include non-alcoholic fatty liver disease (NAFLD), alcohol-related liver disease (ALD), viral hepatitis, and drug-induced liver injury (DILI).[1]

EPIDEMIOLOGY

Between 10% and 21.7% of liver function panels have at least one abnormal result.[1] Abnormal liver function tests are often not investigated or are incompletely evaluated in a primary care setting[2] and commonly with an extended period before evaluation.[3]

---

[a] Department of Gastroenterology, MedStar Georgetown University Hospital, 3800 Reservoir Road Northwest, Washington, DC 20007, USA; [b] Baltimore, MD, USA; [c] Department of Family Medicine, MedStar Georgetown University, 3800 Reservoir Road Northwest, Washington, DC 20007, USA
* Corresponding author.
E-mail address: jessica.j.rosenberg@gunet.georgetown.edu

Prim Care Clin Office Pract 50 (2023) 363–376
https://doi.org/10.1016/j.pop.2023.03.007
0095-4543/23/© 2023 Elsevier Inc. All rights reserved.

NAFLD: In a primary care cohort of over 1000 patients with incidentally diagnosed abnormal liver tests, NAFLD was the underlying abnormality in 26% of cases.[4] Most US studies report an overall 10% to 35% prevalence rate of NAFLD,[5] although this depends on the study population; for example, the prevalence of NAFLD is 80% to 90% in obese adults, 30% to 50% in patients with diabetes mellitus, 90% or more in patients with hyperlipidemia.

NAFLD is the leading cause of chronic liver disease in the United States, accounting for 75% of all chronic liver diseases.[6]

Alcohol-ALD: includes a variety of clinical disorders: steatosis, alcohol-associated steatohepatitis, alcoholic hepatitis, and alcohol-related cirrhosis. ALD is a major cause of liver disease in the United States and can also contribute to the progression of chronic viral hepatitis, NAFLD, iron overload, and other liver diseases.

The prevalence of alcohol-related fatty liver is 4.3% in the United States.[7] However, ALD accounts for up to 48% of cirrhosis-associated deaths in the United States,[8] and ALD has now become the leading indication for liver transplantation in the United States.

VIRAL HEPATITIS

- Hepatitis C: Hepatitis C virus (HCV) infection is the most reported bloodborne infection in the United States.[9] There are an estimated 2.4 million individuals (1.0% of the adult population) in the United States with active hepatitis C infection; 57,500 new cases are estimated to occur annually, and new cases are more likely to occur in men, persons between the ages of 30 and 39, and non-Hispanic White individuals.[9]
- Hepatitis B: The prevalence of hepatitis B surface antigen (HBsAg) positivity in the United States is estimated to be 2.2 million people. Of these, 1.32 million are foreign born with 58% immigrating from high or intermediate endemic areas of Asia.[10]
- Hepatitis A: There are an estimated 24,900 new cases of hepatitis A annually in the United States.[9] Since 2016, 37 states have had either active or recent hepatitis A outbreaks.[11]

Numerous other viruses are known to cause liver inflammation, including

- Epstein-Barr virus
- Herpes simplex virus, and
- Cytomegalovirus

DILI may present with asymptomatic elevations in liver biochemistries. The diagnosis is challenging, and at this time, remains a diagnosis of exclusion. The incidence of DILI in population-based studies has been reported to be 2.7 to 19 per 100,000 people a year.[12]

Less common causes of abnormal liver testing include less common liver diseases such as autoimmune hepatitis, primary biliary cholangitis (PBC), primary sclerosing cholangitis (PSC), and even more rarely Wilson's disease, and alpha-1 antitrypsin deficiency.

PATHOPHYSIOLOGY

The aminotransferases (formerly called transaminases) AST and ALT can be increased due to any process that leads to loss of hepatocyte membrane integrity or necrosis.[13] AST is present in the liver and other organs including cardiac muscle, skeletal muscle, kidney, and brain. ALT, however, is present primarily in the liver, and is a more specific marker of hepatocellular cell injury. Other diseases associated with elevated ALT and AST include musculoskeletal disorders such as polymyositis as well as acute myocardial infarction and hypothyroidism.

In adults, the normal range of ALT levels is approximately 29 to 33 units/L for men and 19 to 25 units/L for women.[14] Despite this, many laboratories use higher upper limit of normal values as high as 55 unit/L for ALT, which may result in a missed opportunity for detection of chronic liver diseases.

ALP is found in hepatocytes as well as in bone, placenta, intestine, and kidney. It can become elevated with obstruction of the bile ducts.[15] Elevation of ALP is not specific to the liver and can be seen in myriad processes.[16]

Bilirubin is the end result of heme catabolism. Bilirubin is conjugated in the liver to bilirubin glucuronide (reported as direct bilirubin), rendering it water-soluble; it is then excreted in bile where it is converted by bacteria in the colon to urobilinogen, which is subsequently excreted in the urine and stool. An increase in conjugated bilirubin is due to decreased excretion into the bile ductules or leakage from hepatocytes into the serum.

The liver is the predominant site of serum protein production, including albumin and coagulation factors. The most used tests to assess the synthetic capacity of the liver are serum albumin and PT.

Albumin is a protein that is made only in the liver. Hypoalbuminemia can indicate hepatic synthetic dysfunction, although albumin concentrations are reduced in other scenarios including sepsis, nephrotic syndrome, malnutrition, and gastrointestinal protein loss.[17]

PT measures the rate of conversion of prothrombin to thrombin. PT requires factors II, V, VII, and X, and fibrinogen, which are also made in the liver. A prolonged PT is not specific for liver disease, and may otherwise indicate treatment with warfarin, consumptive coagulopathy, or Vitamin K deficiency.[18]

Clinical Presentation

It is a common clinical scenario to encounter elevated liver enzymes in an asymptomatic patient.[19]

See **Table 1** for a summary of typical laboratory findings for common causes of abnormal liver chemistries.

NON-ALCOHOLIC FATTY LIVER DISEASE

Patients with NAFLD are frequently asymptomatic, presenting with characteristics common to metabolic syndromes such as insulin resistance, abdominal obesity,

Table 1	
Overview of etiologies and associated treatment of abnormal liver tests	
Etiology	**Treatment**
NAFLD	Diet, exercise, weight loss, blood glucose control (if diabetes present), reduction in heavy alcohol use
ALD	Reducing alcohol intake
Hepatitis A	Supportive care
Hepatitis B	Acute: supportive care; Chronic: nucleos(t)ide analogs, ± interferon
Hepatitis C	Direct acting antiviral medications
DILI	Withdrawal of offending agent, agent-specific treatment if available (eg, NAC for acetaminophen)

hypertension, and dyslipidemia.[20] In asymptomatic patients with NAFLD, lab abnormalities can include transaminase elevations between two to five times the upper limit of normal and a ratio under 1.

Patients with nonalcoholic steatohepatitis (NASH) may present with additional nonspecific findings such as.

- Malaise
- Fatigue, and
- Abdominal discomfort in the right upper quadrant[21]

Advanced disease and ongoing fibrotic response to hepatic inflammation can eventually lead to cirrhosis with its associated stigmata.

ALCOHOL-RELATED LIVER DISEASE

ALD includes a spectrum of liver disorders consisting of alcohol-associated steatosis, alcoholic hepatitis, steatohepatitis, and cirrhosis.

Patients with alcohol-associated fatty liver are often asymptomatic. Patients with alcoholic hepatitis typically present with jaundice, and patients who have developed cirrhosis may have peripheral stigmata of liver disease or signs of hepatic decompensation. Accordingly, physical examination findings in patients with ALD range from normal to evidence of cirrhosis with hepatic decompensation.

When laboratory abnormalities are present, they typically include a mild to moderate elevation of AST and ALT, with the classic finding of AST:ALT ratio >1 (and often >2).

VIRAL HEPATITIS
Hepatitis C

Acute HCV infection generally refers to the first 6 months of HCV infection following presumed HCV exposure.[22] Most patients with acute infection with HCV do not have any symptoms, although they can less commonly have anorexia, malaise, right upper quadrant pain, or jaundice.[23] During the acute phase, ALT levels rise, peaking at 10 to 20 times the upper limit of normal after 2 to 3 months of infection. Normalization of these levels may occur and may be followed later by recurring elevation, indicating chronic disease.[24]

A portion (15%–45%) of patients infected with HCV will spontaneously clear the virus. Progression to chronic infection is characterized by the persistence of ribonucleic acid (RNA) 6 months after initial exposure.

Among patients with chronic hepatitis C infection, the most commonly reported symptoms are

- Fatigue
- Irritability
- Depression, and
- Abdominal pain.[25]

Extrahepatic diseases can be seen, such as mixed cryoglobulinemia and dermatologic conditions.

Approximately 5% to 30% of patients with chronic HCV infection develop cirrhosis over a 20- to 30-year time period.[26]

Hepatitis B

Acute hepatitis B virus (HBV) symptoms include

- Jaundice

- Anorexia
- Headaches
- Malaise
- And gastrointestinal symptoms such as nausea, vomiting, diarrhea, and abdominal pain.

Liver enzyme abnormalities are marked by significant elevations in transaminases up to 1000 to 2000 units/L, typically with AST higher than ALT. Elevations in PT are also seen.

Transaminase elevations can improve in 1 to 4 months for patients who clear HBV.

Chronic hepatitis B infection Is generally characterized into four phases (immune-tolerant, HBeAg-positive immune active, inactive, and HBeAg-negative immune reactivation phase), which account for viral replication and associated immune response as reflected by ALT, serological findings, and liver histology.

Hepatitis A

Infection may be asymptomatic, or associated with

- Abdominal pain
- Nausea and vomiting
- Malaise
- Jaundice, and
- Hepatomegaly.

Unusual presentations include relapsing hepatitis, prolonged cholestasis, or acute liver failure.[27] Associated lab abnormalities include transaminitis >1000 with a predominance of ALT, serum bilirubin that peaks under 10 mg/dL, and alkaline phosphatase elevations >400 U/L.[28] Transaminase elevations generally peak after 1 month.

Drug-Induced Liver Injury

DILI can be categorized as either intrinsic (predictably causes liver injury at certain high doses, eg, acetaminophen), or more commonly, idiosyncratic (with an inconsistent relationship to dose and variable laboratory/clinical presentation).

Idiosyncratic DILI can have multiple presentations. Often asymptomatic elevations in liver chemistries are seen. Those who develop symptoms can have

- Weakness
- Fever
- Nausea and vomiting
- Right upper quadrant pain, and
- Jaundice.[29]
  Severe cases can result in progression to chronic hepatitis or even acute liver failure.

The most common clinical presentations of DILI are hepatocellular, cholestatic, and mixed, with a pattern of injury defined using the R value (**Fig. 1**).

The outcomes of idiosyncratic DILI are favorable, with only about 10% reaching the threshold of acute liver failure and fewer than 20% developing chronic liver injury.[30]

Diagnosis

Initial work-up of any abnormal liver-related tests should first involve repeating the initial test.

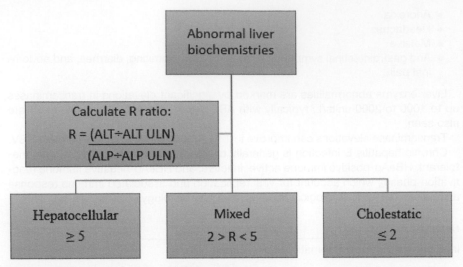

Fig. 1. Determining the pattern of liver injury.

The magnitude and pattern of initial liver test elevations, in addition to clinical presentation and risk factors informed by a thorough history and physical exam, should guide initial labs, imaging, and referrals.

Testing abnormalities can adhere to several patterns depending on etiology; calculation of the R ratio can help classify patterns into hepatocellular, mixed, or cholestatic liver injury (see **Fig. 1**).[14] In individuals with suspected hepatocellular or mixed DILI, acute viral hepatitis (A, B, and C) and autoimmune hepatitis should be excluded with standard serologies and HCV-RNA testing. Second-line testing can include testing for other viruses hepatitis E virus, cytomegalovirus, Ebstein Barr virus, or herpes simplex virus (HEV, CMV, EBV, or HSV), ceruloplasmin to test for Wilson's disease, and abdominal imaging to evaluate for Budd-Chiari syndrome when clinically appropriate.

If it is cholestatic injury, hepatobiliary imaging should be performed to evaluate for biliary tract pathology and PBC should be tested for. Second-line testing may include more invasive testing such as endoscopic retrograde cholangiopancreatography (ERCP).[30]

A borderline AST and/or ALT elevation is defined as <2X upper limit of normal (ULN), a mild AST and/or ALT elevation as 2–5X ULN, moderate AST and/or ALT elevation 5–15X ULN, severe AST and/or ALT elevation >15X ULN, and massive AST and/or ALT >10,000 IU/L. See **Fig. 2** for an initial work-up of borderline, mild, and moderate AST and ALT elevations.[14]

Non-alcoholic fatty liver disease the diagnosis of NAFLD is often made incidentally or as part of the work-up for patients presenting with hepatomegaly and mild transaminase elevations.[31]

The diagnosis of NAFLD requires the presence of steatosis by imaging or histology and lack of significant alcohol consumption or other competing etiologies for steatosis or chronic liver disease.

The primary abnormality in NAFLD is mild to moderately elevated serum aminotransferases, although liver enzymes can be normal. When elevated, the AST and ALT are usually below 300 IU/L, with an AST to ALT ratio of less than 1. Alkaline phosphatase may be elevated to two to three times the upper limit of normal.

There can be laboratory abnormalities in patients with NAFLD that do not always reflect the presence of another liver disease. For example, mildly elevated serum

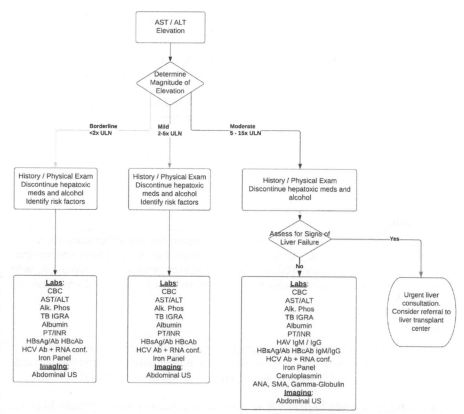

Fig. 2. Initial diagnostics for elevated AST and ALT. (*Adapted from* Kwo PY, Cohen SM, Lim JK. ACG Clinical Guideline: Evaluation of Abnormal Liver Chemistries. Am J Gastroenterol. 2017;112(1):18-35.)

ferritin is a common feature of NAFLD that does not necessarily indicate hepatic iron overload. Low titers of serum autoantibodies, particularly antismooth muscle and antinuclear antibodies, are common.

Radiographic findings consistent with NAFLD include increased echogenicity on ultrasound, decreased hepatic attenuation on CT, and increased fat signal on MRI.

In general, biopsy should be performed in those who would benefit the most from diagnosis, therapeutic guidance, and prognostic information, for example, such as in patients who have competing etiologies for hepatic steatosis, and when the presence and/or severity of coexisting chronic liver diseases (CLDs) cannot be excluded without a liver biopsy.

Finally, the initial evaluation of patients with suspected NAFLD should include consideration of the presence of commonly associated comorbidities such as obesity, dyslipidemia, diabetes, hypothyroidism, polycystic ovary syndrome, and sleep apnea.[32]

Alcohol-Related Liver Disease

In the primary care setting, alcohol-ALD should be suspected in patients with a history of significant alcohol use who present with abnormal aminotransferases, hepatomegaly, or radiographic imaging suggesting hepatic steatosis, fibrosis, or cirrhosis.

The pattern of liver injury associated with alcoholic liver injury is an AST:ALT ratio of at least 2:1, with values of AST or ALT rarely exceeding 300 IU/L.[33]

Clinical and laboratory features are typically sufficient for establishing the diagnosis of ALD in a patient with a history of excessive alcohol use, given that the patient does not have risk factors for other causes of liver disease and a negative work-up for other common causes of liver disease.

The definition of significant alcohol consumption has been suggested as >210 g of alcohol per week in men and >140 g per week in women.[34] Primary care providers should screen for alcohol use with a single question: "How many times in the past year have you had five (four for women) or more drinks in a day?" If the patient reports even a single episode, additional testing is recommended.[35]

Confirmation of diagnosis requires exclusion of alternative causes of hepatitis, including infectious, metabolic, and DILI.

Viral Hepatitis

The diagnosis of infectious hepatitis involves serologic testing, often confirmed with detection of viral nucleic acid. Acute hepatitis typically can present with aminotransferase levels measured in the 1000s. Chronic hepatitis varies in presentation, with aminotransferase levels typically elevated to no more than 2 times to 10 times the upper limit of normal.[36]

Hepatitis B

Hepatitis B status involves three serologic tests: HBsAg, indicative of hepatitis B infection; the hepatitis B core antibody total, indicative of prior exposure; and the hepatitis B surface antibody, which signals either natural or vaccine-mediated immunity to infection.[37]

The diagnosis of acute hepatitis B is made by a positive immunoglobulin M (IgM), hepatitis B core antibody (hepatitis B core antibody IgM), and HBsAg in the setting of an acute hepatitis.

The diagnosis of chronic hepatitis B (CHB) is based upon the persistence of HBsAg for greater than 6 months. Notably, serum HBV deoxyribonucleic acid (DNA) can range from undetectable to more than 1 billion IU/mL. Laboratory tests should include assessment of liver disease activity and function, markers of HBV replication, and tests for coinfection (HCV, hepatitis delta virus [HDV], or HIV).[38] An evaluation for fibrosis and/or cirrhosis should be performed as well, using abdominal ultrasound, elastography, or serum fibrosis assessments, for example, the online FIB-4 calculator.

Hepatitis C

The initial evaluation of a patient with suspected HCV exposure or infection begins with antibody testing.[39] A positive HCV-antibody test can indicate a current/active HCV infection, a past resolved infection, or a false-positive result. Diagnosis to confirm the active infection is confirmed with HCV-RNA testing, which is completed reflexively in most settings.

In a patient with a known prior HCV infection that has previously cleared either spontaneously or due to treatment, HCV-RNA testing must be done instead of antibody testing, as HCV-antibody is expected to remain positive.

Acute HCV infection is defined as the first 6 months of infection and is marked by elevations in HCV-RNA 2 to 3 weeks after exposure, and the development of antibodies in 2 to 3 months.

Hepatitis A

Diagnosis of hepatitis A virus (HAV) infection is confirmed by serologic evidence of a recent infection, with detection of immunoglobulin G (IgM) antibodies against HAV. IgM antibodies typically peak about a month after exposure and can persist for up to a year. IgG response typically follows IgM response after 1 week, and usually persists indefinitely.

Drug-Induced Liver Injury

The diagnosis of DILI can be challenging, and DILI remains a diagnosis of exclusion. A thorough history of medication exposure is crucial when there is suspicion of drug-related hepatotoxicity. Patients should be asked about the most commonly associated drugs, which include antibiotics and antiepileptic medications. Amoxicillin-clavulanate continues to be the most commonly implicated drug in most Western countries. The use of herbal and dietary supplements should be discussed, and a thorough timeline of doses and usage should be elicited.

DILI can present with hepatocellular, cholestatic, or mixed injury pattern. The online resource *LiverTox* contains information on more than 1200 agents and their possible association with DILI as well as typical patterns of injury.[40] The overwhelmingly most common agent involved in DILI is acetaminophen. Among non-acetaminophen-related agents, the next most commonly observed agents in a prospective national cohort in the United States are

- Amoxicillin-clavulanate
- Isoniazid
- Nitrofurantoin
- Sulfamethoxazole/trimethoprim, and
- Minocycline

Among classes of medications, antimicrobials are the most common causative agent, followed by herbal and dietary supplements, cardiovascular agents, central nervous system agents, and anti-neoplastic agents.[41]

A liver biopsy should be considered when there is suspicion for possible autoimmune hepatitis, or if ongoing rise in liver enzymes despite stopping the suspected agent, or if liver abnormalities persist beyond 180 days.

Scoring systems such as the Roussel Uclaf Causality Assessment Method (RUCAM) can be used to help determine the causality of a suspected agent.

If uncertainty persists after thorough history and evaluation for competing etiologies, patients should be referred to a liver specialist for further evaluation.

Management

Non-alcoholic fatty liver disease

The management of NAFLD includes treating not only liver disease, but also the associated metabolic comorbidities.

Weight loss through diet and exercise is the primary therapy for most patients with NAFLD. Weight loss of 7% to 10% is needed to improve most of the histopathological features of NASH, including fibrosis.[42] More research is needed regarding whether specific diets, such as the Mediterranean diet, improve outcomes. Pharmacologic therapy for weight loss purposes in patients who fail to achieve their goals through diet and exercise alone can also be used.

Bariatric surgery is an option for those who are unable to achieve sustained weight loss through diet and exercise. The primary care clinic is the ideal setting to discuss the risks and benefits associated with bariatric surgery and provide referrals if needed.[43]

Pharmacological treatments aimed primarily at improving liver disease should generally be limited to those with biopsy-proven NASH and fibrosis.[32] Pioglitazone improves liver histology in patients with and without type 2 diabetes mellitus (T2DM) with biopsy-proven NASH. Vitamin E administered at a daily dose of 800 IU/day improves liver histology in nondiabetic adults with biopsy-proven NASH.

Finally, patients should be counseled on the risks of alcohol use, with heavy alcohol use associated with disease progression.[44] Risk of disease progression with non-heavy consumption of alcohol by individuals with NAFLD is not yet known. Vaccination for hepatitis A virus and hepatitis B virus should be given if applicable. Management of patients with NAFLD and diabetes includes optimization of blood glucose control. Most patients with NAFLD and hyperlipidemia may benefit from lipid-lowering therapy.

Alcohol-related liver disease the treatment of ALD is based on cessation of alcohol intake. The role of the primary care physician is critical to ensure appropriate coordination of both psychosocial and clinical interventions.

Historically, glucocorticoids and pentoxifylline have been components of the management of ALD. However, reviews of existing literature have found weak evidence supporting any benefits from their use.[45] When weighed against increased risk of infection, the primary care provider should use glucocorticoids with caution.

VIRAL HEPATITIS
Hepatitis B

Treatment of acute HBV is typically supportive, although patients with severe or prolonged disease, or risk factors of severe disease such as immunocompromised state or concomitant HCV infection should be considered for treatment.

In the primary care setting, the foundations of chronic hepatitis B management are based on counseling and prevention of transmission of HBV to others. Patients should be counseled on long-term implications of chronic infection, such as cirrhosis and hepatocellular carcinoma (HCC). They should be advised to avoid or limit alcohol use, and to optimize body weight to prevent development of hepatic steatosis.

Patients should also be educated on how to prevent transmission of HBV to others (eg, cover cuts and scratches, use condoms, and avoid sharing razors or injection equipment).

Hepatitis B immune globulin and vaccine can be provided to all household and sexual contacts who cannot confirm immunity to HBV.

Individuals confirmed to have chronic hepatitis B should be referred to physicians with expertise in its management. Treatment of chronic HBV typically includes PegIFN or nucleos(t)ide analogs.

Primary care providers should be aware of the indications for HCC surveillance, which include all patients with cirrhosis, or other high-risk patients such as African Americans or older Asian Americans. HCC surveillance can be performed in the primary care setting with liver ultrasound every 6 months.

Hepatitis C

Antiviral treatment is strongly recommended for all adults with acute or chronic HCV infection, except for those with short life expectancy. HCV treatment can be effectively provided in the primary care setting, and there are simplified treatment algorithms designed to be used by any health care provider knowledgeable about HCV disease and treatment.[39]

Treatment of chronic HCV with direct acting antiviral medications (DAAs) is highly efficacious. The simplified regimen depends on whether or not cirrhosis is present in a treatment-naïve adult.

A post-treatment assessment of cure (sustained virologic response [SVR]) with HCV-RNA and AST and ALT testing should be completed 12 weeks after completion of treatment. Patients who fail initial treatment should be evaluated by a specialist for retreatment.

Hepatitis A

Treatment is supportive. In the rare event of fulminant liver failure, the patient must be immediately referred to a transplant center.

DRUG-INDUCED LIVER INJURY

Suspected agents in individuals with suspected DILI should be immediately stopped.

Specific treatments are rare, such as L-carnitine for valproic acid overdoses and N-acetylcysteine (NAC) for acetaminophen poisoning. There are no definitive therapies for idiosyncratic DILI.[30]

The data are mixed regarding the use of corticosteroid therapy in patients with DILI. They should be considered in patients with DILI who have autoimmune hepatitis-like features.

Primary care providers can assist with prevention of DILI by undertaking regular medical reconciliations, ensuring that they specifically ask patients to report use of herbal and dietary supplements.

Patients with DILI who develop progressive jaundice or acute liver failure should be referred to a liver transplantation center.

WHEN TO REFER TO GASTROENTEROLOGY (GI)

In general, the decision of when to refer to a gastroenterologist depends both on clinical context and the magnitude of elevation of liver-associated enzymes.

- Patients with marked elevations of transaminases (eg, ALT >1,000 U/L).
- Persistent elevation of liver enzymes (eg, >2 times upper limit of normal for AST, ALT or greater than 1.5 times upper limit of normal for alkaline phosphatase) that is unexplained.
- Patients with evidence of a high risk of advanced fibrosis or cirrhosis based on imaging or other noninvasive scoring systems should be referred to a liver specialist.
- Patients with DILI who develop progressive jaundice with or without coagulopathy should be referred to a liver transplantation center.

CLINICS CARE POINTS

- NAFLD is the leading cause of chronic liver disease in the United States, accounting for 75% of all chronic liver diseases.
- The gold standard for determining the presence of liver fibrosis or cirrhosis is a liver biopsy; however, this can more typically be assessed using various noninvasive scoring systems (eg, Fibrosis-4 [FIB-4] index) or the use of transient elastography.
- ALD has now become the leading indication for liver transplantation in the United States. Primary care providers should screen all patients for alcohol use.

- Antiviral treatment is recommended for all adults with acute or chronic HCV infection, except for those with short life expectancy. HCV treatment can be effectively provided in the primary care setting.

REFERENCES

1. Radcke S, Dillon JF, Murray AL. A systematic review of the prevalence of mildly abnormal liver function tests and associated health outcomes. Eur J Gastroenterol Hepatol 2015;27(1):1–7.
2. Sherwood P, Lyburn I, Brown S, et al. How are abnormal results for liver function tests dealt with in primary care? Audit of yield and impact. BMJ 2001;322(7281): 276–8.
3. Schreiner AD, Mauldin PD, Moran WP, et al. Assessing the Burden of Abnormal LFTs and the Role of the Electronic Health Record: A Retrospective Study. Am J Med Sci 2018;355(6):537–43.
4. Armstrong MJ, Houlihan DD, Bentham L, et al. Presence and severity of non-alcoholic fatty liver disease in a large prospective primary care cohort. J Histotechnol 2012;56(1):234–40.
5. Vernon G, Baranova A, Younossi ZM. Systematic review: the epidemiology and natural history of non-alcoholic fatty liver disease and non-alcoholic steatohepatitis in adults. Aliment Pharmacol Ther 2011;34(3):274–85.
6. Wong RJ, Liu B, Bhukel T. Significant burden of nonalcoholic fatty liver disease with advanced fibrosis in the US: a cross-sectional analysis of 2011-2014 National Health and Nutrition Examination Survey. Aliment Pharmacol Ther 2017; 46:974–80.
7. Wong T, Dang K, Ladhani S, et al. Prevalence of alcoholic fatty liver disease among adults in the United States. JAMA 2019;321:1723–5.
8. Yoon YH and Chen CM, *Surveillance Report #105. Liver cirrhosis mortality in the United States: national, state, and regional trends, 2000–2013, Surveillance Report #105. Liver cirrhosis mortality in the United States: national, state, and regional trends, 2000–2013*, 2016, National Institute on Alcohol Abuse and Alcoholism (NIAAA); Bethesda (MD), Available at: http://pubs.niaaa.nih.gov/publications/Surveillanc e105/Cirr13.pd, Accessed February 2023.
9. Centers for Disease Control and Prevention. 2019 Viral Hepatitis Surveillance Report. Available at: https://www.cdc.gov/hepatitis/statistics/SurveillanceRpts. htm. Published July 2021. Accessed October 2022.
10. Kowdley KV, Wang CC, Welch S, et al. Prevalence of chronic hepatitis B among foreign-born persons living in the United States by country of origin. Hepatology 2012;56:422–33.
11. Available at: https://www.cdc.gov/hepatitis/outbreaks/2017March-HepatitisA. htm.
12. Björnsson ES. Epidemiology, predisposing factors, and outcomes of drug-induced liver injury. Clin Liver Dis 2020;24(1):1–10.
13. Moriles KE, Azer SA. Alanine amino transferase. [Updated 2022 Dec 10]. In: StatPearls Internet. Treasure Island (FL): StatPearls Publishing; 2023. Available at: https://www.ncbi.nlm.nih.gov/books/NBK559278/.
14. Kwo PY, Cohen SM, Lim JK. ACG clinical guideline: evaluation of abnormal liver chemistries. Am J Gastroenterol 2017;112(1):18–35.
15. Vroon DH, Israili Z. Alkaline phosphatase and gamma glutamyltransferase. In: Walker HK, Hall WD, Hurst JW, editors. Clinical methods: the history, physical,

and laboratory examinations. 3rd edition. Boston: Butterworths; 1990. p. 494–5. Chapter 100. Available at: https://www.ncbi.nlm.nih.gov/books/NBK203/If needed. Chapter 100. Available at:.

16. Lowe D. Sanvictores T. John S. Alkaline Phosphatase. Updated 2022 Aug 8. In: StatPearls Internet. Treasure Island (FL): StatPearls Publishing; 2022 Jan-. Available at: https://www.ncbi.nlm.nih.gov/books/NBK459201/.

17. Newsome PN, Cramb R, Davison SM, et al. Guidelines on the management of abnormal liver blood tests. Gut 2018;67:6–19.

18. Lala V. Goyal A. Minter DA. Liver Function Tests. Updated 2022 Mar 19. In: StatPearls Internet. Treasure Island (FL): StatPearls Publishing; 2022 Jan-. Available at: https://www.ncbi.nlm.nih.gov/books/NBK482489/.

19. Ioannou GN, Boyko EJ, Lee SP. The prevalence and predictors of elevated serum aminotransferase activity in the United States in 1999–2002. Am J Gastroenterol 2006;101:76–82.

20. Ma J, Hwang SJ, Pedley A, et al. "Bi-directional analysis between fatty liver and cardiovascular disease risk factors.". J Hepatol 2017;66(2):390–7.

21. Bacon BR, Farahvash MJ, Janney CG, et al. "Nonalcoholic steatohepatitis: an expanded clinical entity.". Gastroenterology 1994;107(4):1103–9.

22. Blackard JT, Shata MT, Shire NJ, et al. Acute hepatitis C virus infection: a chronic problem. Hepatology 2008;47(1):321–31 [Erratum in: Hepatology. 2008 Feb;47(2):769].

23. Marcellin P. "Hepatitis C: the clinical spectrum of the disease.". J Hepatol 1999; 31:9–16.

24. Bonkovsky HL, Mehta S. Hepatitis C: a review and update. J Am Acad Dermatol 2001;44(2):159–82.

25. Lang CA, Conrad S, Garrett L, et al. Symptom prevalence and clustering of symptoms in people living with chronic hepatitis C infection. J Pain Symptom Manage 2006;31(4):335–44.

26. Thein HH, Yi Q, Dore GJ, et al. Estimation of stage-specific fibrosis progression rates in chronic hepatitis C virus infection: a meta-analysis and meta-regression. Hepatology 2008;48:418–31.

27. Abutaleb A, Kottilil S, Hepatitis A. Epidemiology, natural history, unusual clinical manifestations, and prevention. Gastroenterol Clin North Am 2020;49(2):191–9.

28. Tong MJ, el-Farra NS, Grew MI. Clinical manifestations of hepatitis a: recent experience in a community teaching hospital. J Infect Dis 1995;1(171 Suppl):S15–8.

29. Lu RJ, Zhang Y, Tang FL, et al. Clinical characteristics of drug-induced liver injury and related risk factors. Exp Ther Med 2016;12(4):2606–16.

30. Chalasani NP, Maddur H, Russo MW, et al. Practice parameters committee of the american college of gastroenterology. ACG clinical guideline: diagnosis and management of idiosyncratic drug-induced liver injury. Am J Gastroenterol 2021;116(5):878–98.

31. Sangeetha A, Prabhuswamy KM. "Prevalence and profile of non-alcoholic fatty liver disease among adults undergoing master health checkup, a Hospital Based Cross Sectional Study.". International Journal of Contemporary Medical Research 2019;6(no. 8). https://doi.org/10.21276/ijcmr.2019.6.8.52.

32. Chalasani N, Younossi Z, Lavine JE, et al. The diagnosis and management of nonalcoholic fatty liver disease: practice guidance from the american association for the study of liver diseases. Hepatology 2018;67(1):328–57.

33. Kawachi I, Robinson GM, Stace NH. A combination of raised serum AST: ALT ratio and erythrocyte mean cell volume level detects excessive alcohol consumption. N Z Med J 1990;103(887):145–8.

34. Chalasani N, Younossi Z, Lavine JE, et al. The diagnosis and management of non-alcoholic fatty liver disease: practice guideline by the american association for the study of liver diseases, american college of gastroenterology, and the american gastroenterological association. Hepatology 2012;55(6):2005–23.
35. Saunders JB, Aasland OG, Babor TF, et al. Development of the Alcohol Use Disorders Identification Test (AUDIT): WHO collaborative project on early detection of persons with harmful alcohol consumption—II. Addiction 1993;88:791–804.
36. Giannini EG, Testa R, Savarino V. Liver enzyme alteration: a guide for clinicians. CMAJ (Can Med Assoc J) 2005;172(3):367–79.
37. Lok AS, McMahon BJ. Chronic hepatitis B: update 2009. Hepatology 2009;50(3):661–2.
38. Terrault NA, Lok ASF, McMahon BJ, et al. Update on prevention, diagnosis, and treatment of chronic hepatitis B: AASLD 2018 hepatitis B guidance. Hepatology 2018;67(4):1560–99.
39. Ghany MG, Morgan TR. AASLD-IDSA Hepatitis C Guidance Panel. Hepatitis C Guidance 2019 Update: american association for the study of liver diseases-infectious diseases society of america recommendations for testing, managing, and treating Hepatitis C virus infection. Hepatology 2020;71(2):686–721.
40. LiverTox: clinical and research information on drug-induced liver injury. Bethesda, MD: NIDDK; 2012.
41. Chalasani N, Bonkovsky HL, Fontana R, et al. United States drug induced liver injury network. features and outcomes of 899 patients with drug-induced liver injury: The DILIN Prospective Study. Gastroenterology 2015;148(7):1340–52.e7.
42. Musso G, Cassader M, Rosina F, et al. "Impact of Current Treatments on Liver Disease, Glucose Metabolism and Cardiovascular Risk in Non-Alcoholic Fatty Liver Disease (NAFLD): a systematic review and meta-analysis of randomised trials.". Diabetologia 2012;55(4):885–904.
43. Lee Y, Doumouras AG, Yu J, et al. "Complete resolution of nonalcoholic fatty liver disease after bariatric surgery: a systematic review and meta-analysis.". Clin Gastroenterol Hepatol 2019;17(6). https://doi.org/10.1016/j.cgh.2018.10.017.
44. Ekstedt M, Franzén LE, Holmqvist M, et al. Alcohol consumption is associated with progression of hepatic fibrosis in non-alcoholic fatty liver disease. Scand J Gastroenterol 2009;44(3):366–74.
45. Pavlov CS, Varganova DL, Casazza G, et al. Glucocorticosteroids for people with alcoholic hepatitis. Cochrane Database Syst Rev 2019;(4):CD001511. https://doi.org/10.1002/14651858.CD001511.pub4.

Diseases of the Gallbladder and Biliary Tree

Seth Anthony Politano, DO[a],*, Nida Hamiduzzaman, MD[b], Dalal Alhaqqan, MBBCh[c]

KEYWORDS

- Gallbladder • Biliary • Jaundice • Cholecystitis • Gallstones • Choledocholithiasis
- Cysts • Polyps

KEY POINTS

- Diseases of the gallbladder have a wide array of clinical presentations, with some requiring urgent intervention, and others monitoring.
- In the setting of gallstone disease, the presence of inflammatory markers, liver enzyme elevation, or hemodynamic instability warrants urgent referral.
- Management of biliary cysts is dependent on type classification, but referral should be sought in almost all cases, especially when there is ductal dilation.
- Gallbladder polyps that are 1 cm or greater in size should undergo cholecystectomy because of the increased risk of developing gallbladder cancer.

INTRODUCTION

Diseases of the biliary system are varied and range from an uncomplicated benign disease to acute emergencies and chronic conditions. The gallbladder plays a role in storage, digestion, and absorption. Bile produced by the liver is stored in the gallbladder, moving from the hepatic ducts through the cystic duct of the gallbladder for storage. Production of cholecystokinin after meal ingestion signals the gallbladder to contract. Bile flows from the gallbladder, through the common bile duct (CBD), to join the pancreatic duct and is eventually released into the small intestine. This bile aids in digestion and absorption of fat. The bile also serves as a means via which bilirubin is removed from the body. The gallbladder is not necessary for digestion, however, and patients after cholecystectomy are usually asymptomatic. There are a few exceptions of postcholecystectomy patients having indigestion, bloating, diarrhea, and flatulence.

---

[a] College of Osteopathic Medicine of the Pacific, Western University of Health Sciences, Pomona, CA, USA; [b] Division of GHPGIM, Keck School of Medicine of USC, Los Angeles, CA, USA; [c] Division of Gastroenterology and Hepatology, MedStar Georgetown University Hospital, Washington, DC, USA
* Corresponding author. Western U, College of Osteopathic Medicine of the Pacific, 309 E 2nd Street, Pomona, CA 91766.
E-mail address: Docsethp@yahoo.com

Prim Care Clin Office Pract 50 (2023) 377–390
https://doi.org/10.1016/j.pop.2023.03.004
0095-4543/23/© 2023 Elsevier Inc. All rights reserved.

Cholelithiasis and Cholecystitis

Prevalence/incidence

Gallstones in the gallbladder (cholelithiasis) affect approximately 10% to 15% of the US population although a majority are asymptomatic. Only about 20% of patients with cholelithiasis will develop any symptoms or complications, including cholecystitis, cholangitis, or pancreatitis.[1] Another complication, albeit rare, is gallstone ileus. Out of these complications, cholecystitis is the most common one, seen in approximately 10% of symptomatic patients.

Gallstones are most prevalent in Native Americans of North and South America, followed by Mexican Americans, White Americans, Black Americans, and Asian Americans. In addition, women more commonly have gallstones than men.[1] Additional risk factors for gallstones are presented in **Box 1** below.

Cholecystitis, or inflammation of the gallbladder, could be due to the presence or absence of gallstones. Acalculous cholecystitis is uncommon, representing 5% to 10% of cases of cholecystitis.[2] It usually results from biliary stasis and is seen in critically ill (septic, ventilated) patients, those with severe burns, on total parenteral nutrition, and in patients with advanced human immunodeficiency virus (HIV).

Pathophysiology

Gallstones (**Fig. 1**) in the Western world are predominantly cholesterol stones, followed by pigmented (calcium bilirubinate) gallstones.[3] Mixed gallstones can also occur.

Cholesterol gallstones can result from increased precipitation of solid crystals in bile and increased secretion of biliary cholesterol by the liver or gallbladder dysmotility. Other causes include slowed intestinal motility and decreased cholesterol absorption by the intestines. In addition, a variety of genetic factors can increase the amount of cholesterol gallstones.[4]

Pigmented, or brown, gallstones in the Eastern world are caused mostly by parasitic infections involving the biliary tree (such as the *Clonorchis* species). In the Western world, chronic inflammation from malignancy or strictures can result in pigmented stones.[1] Another cause of pigmented stones is chronic hemolysis, as seen in sickle cell disease, congenital hemoglobinopathies, autoimmune hemolysis, and red cell membrane disorders such as spherocytosis. Pigmented stones are also the most common stones in patients with cirrhosis.[5]

Box 1
Risk factors for gallstone disease

Risk factors
  Family history
  Genetics
  Age
  Inflammatory bowel disease
  Elevated body mass index
  Diabetes type II
  Dyslipidemia
  Increased alcohol consumption
  Rapid weight loss
  Total parenteral nutrition
  Dietary consumption (red meats, saturated and trans fats)
  Medications (thiazide diuretics, cephalosporins, estrogens, fibrates, somatostatin analogs)
  Solid organ transplantation
  Bariatric surgery

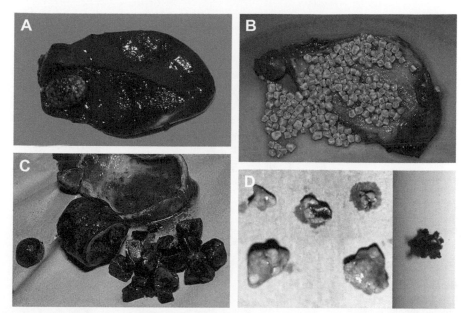

Fig. 1. Different compositions of gallstones. (*A*) Large stone formed by smaller stones in an inflamed gallbladder. (*B*) Multiple stones. (*C*) Large stone. (*D*) Cholesterol stones on left, and pigment stone on right. (*From* Quick CRG, Biers SM, Arulampalam, THA. Chapter 20: Gallstone Diseases and Related Disorders. In: Quick CRG, Biers SM, Arulampalam, THA, eds. Essential Surgery: Problems, Diagnosis and Management. 6th ed. Elsevier; 307-318.)

Cholecystitis results from the blockage and subsequent infection of the gallbladder. *Escherichia coli* is the most common organism.[6] When gas-forming bacteria are involved, emphysematous cholecystitis can occur.[7]

Clinical presentation

Symptomatic cholelithiasis presents with recurrent epigastric and/or right-upper-quadrant pain. The pain lasts up to 6 hours and can radiate to the right shoulder or back. This could be associated with nausea and emesis. The pain can be postprandial or associated with certain dietary intake (fatty, large meals). Belching, indigestion, or dyspepsia can occur.[8] Fever and systemic symptoms are absent. Additional clinical presentations can be seen with complications of cholelithiasis. Gallstone pancreatitis presents with severe mid-epigastric pain that may radiate to the back. Nausea and/or vomiting are present and more severe than with uncomplicated cholelithiasis. Gallstone ileus presents with nausea, vomiting, severe crampy abdominal pain, and distention. Fever can be seen, which could be a sign of concomitant cholecystitis or perforation. A more rare form of gallstone ileus presents with gastric outlet obstruction (**Fig. 2**).

Cholecystitis can present acutely or chronically. Acutely, patients will have right-upper-quadrant pain. This pain is constant and lasts for more than 6 hours. Patients will also have

- Malaise
- Fevers and chills
- Nausea
- Vomiting

Of note, the elderly and diabetics may present atypically, with vague nonspecific symptoms such as fatigue or loss of appetite. Chronic cholecystitis results from

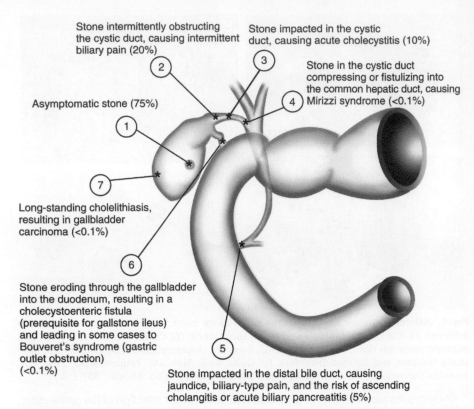

Stone intermittently obstructing the cystic duct, causing intermittent biliary pain (20%)

Stone impacted in the cystic duct, causing acute cholecystitis (10%)

Stone in the cystic duct compressing or fistulizing into the common hepatic duct, causing Mirizzi syndrome (<0.1%)

Asymptomatic stone (75%)

Long-standing cholelithiasis, resulting in gallbladder carcinoma (<0.1%)

Stone eroding through the gallbladder into the duodenum, resulting in a cholecystoenteric fistula (prerequisite for gallstone ileus) and leading in some cases to Bouveret's syndrome (gastric outlet obstruction) (<0.1%)

Stone impacted in the distal bile duct, causing jaundice, biliary-type pain, and the risk of ascending cholangitis or acute biliary pancreatitis (5%)

Fig. 2. Anatomic diagram of gallstone disease locations and complications. (*From* Wang DQH, Afdhal NH. Chapter 65: Gallstone Disease. In: Feldman M, Friedman LS, Brandt LJ, eds. Sleisenger and Fordtran's Gastrointestinal and Liver Disease. 11th ed. Elsevier; 1016-1046.e7.)

subclinical passage of stones. In these cases, symptoms are less severe and last for weeks.[2] This condition has a risk of progression to gallbladder malignancy.

Diagnosis

Laboratory findings with cholelithiasis, even with symptoms, are often normal. Laboratory findings with cholecystitis include leukocytosis with a neutrophil predominance. A left shift may be seen. Lactate levels may be elevated, as well as other inflammatory markers. The liver panel is oftentimes normal. An exception to this is Mirizzi syndrome, where a large, distended gallbladder encroaches the CBD and leads to elevated conjugated hyperbilirubinemia, increased alkaline phosphatase (ALP), and minor elevations in transaminase levels.

The initial radiographic evaluation for cholelithiasis and cholecystitis is an abdominal ultrasound (US). This is cost-effective and safe. Although it has good sensitivity and specificity, results are operator-dependent.[9] Cholecystitis findings include not only the presence of gallstones and/or a distended gallbladder but also gallbladder wall thickening (>4 mm), pericholecystic fluid, and a positive Murphy's sign (pain at the right upper quadrant with insertion of the probe in the area, particular with inspiration).[9] Of note, even though Murphy sign is highly sensitive, it is not very specific. Gas can be seen in the gallbladder with emphysematous cholecystitis.

Computed tomography (CT) scans are not required for diagnostic evaluation of cholelithiasis or cholecystitis. It should be performed only if the diagnosis is in question or additional imaging is needed for another reason. Findings are similar to those seen in ultrasonography.

If patients present with symptoms and laboratory evaluation which is suggestive of cholecystitis, but ultrasonography is negative or unequivocal, cholescintigraphy can be performed. The hepatobiliary iminodiacetic acid (HIDA) scan has reported variability for diagnosis of acute cholecystitis, ranging from 87% to 97% in sensitivity and 79% to 90% in specificity for cholecystitis.[10]

The 2013/2018 Tokyo Guidelines[11] (**Box 2**) define a diagnosis of acute cholecystitis as

Treatment
Patients with cholelithiasis can be managed with nonsteroidal anti-inflammatory drugs for pain. Even after 1 episode of biliary colic, they should be referred for cholecystectomy, which is most often performed laparoscopically.

Cholecystitis should be managed acutely with intravenous fluids and antibiotics in most cases. Antibiotics should cover common organisms that lead to infection, including gram-negative rods and anaerobes. There is increasing prevalence of extended spectrum beta-lactamase–producing organisms,[6] and attention to local resistance patterns, as well as a patient's previous infections, could prompt the use of carbapenems for management. In patients with severe acute cholecystitis, and signs of end-organ damage, enterococcal infections should be considered and covered (ampicillin or vancomycin, and in areas of high vancomycin resistance, linezolid or daptomycin).[6]

Symptomatic management, including pain mediation, antipyretics, as well as antiemetics, can be given as needed. Antibiotics, however, are only temporizing measures, as patients will eventually need a cholecystectomy. This procedure can be performed laparoscopically (preferably), open, or robotically.

In patients that are critically ill, or where surgery poses too high of a risk, a cholecystostomy tube can be placed. Although this does help the disease acutely, recurrent symptoms are common.[2]

When to refer
- Referral to a surgeon should occur with symptomatic cholelithiasis for elective intervention.

Box 2
Tokyo guidelines for diagnosis of cholecystitis

A. Local signs of inflammation include (1) Murphy sign and (2) right upper quadrant (RUQ) mass/pain/tenderness

B. Systemic signs of inflammation: (1) fever, (2) elevated C-reactive protein, (3) elevated white blood cell count

C. Imaging findings characteristic of acute cholecystitis

Suspected diagnosis: 1 item in A + 1 item in B

Definite diagnosis: 1 item in A + 1 item in B + C

Yokoe, M., Takada, T., Strasberg, S.M. et al. New diagnostic criteria and severity assessment of acute cholecystitis in revised Tokyo guidelines. J Hepatobiliary Pancreat Sci 19, 578–585 (2012). https://doi.org/10.1007/s00534-012-0548-0

- Patients with concern for cholecystitis should be evaluated in an inpatient setting/emergency department because of the need for urgent evaluation and the risk of complications if left untreated.

Choledocholithiasis

Prevalence/incidence
Choledocholithiasis describes the presence of gallstones in the biliary tree. It can be further classified into primary and secondary choledocholithiasis. Primary choledocholithiasis refers to the formation of stones within the biliary tree. Secondary choledocholithiasis occurs when gallstones migrate out of the gallbladder and into the biliary tree. Overall, choledocholithiasis occurs in up to 15% of patients that have cholelithiasis and is the most common cause of acute pancreatitis.[12]

Pathophysiology
While the pathophysiology of stone formation is the same as that in cholelithiasis, the prevalence of the type of stone differs with pigmented stones being more common in choledocholithiasis than cholesterol stones in cholelithiasis.[13]

Clinical presentation
Patients usually have a prior history of chronic intermittent abdominal pain that can vary in location. The presentation with choledocholithiasis usually includes right-upper-quadrant colicky pain. They may notice signs of jaundice, as well as nausea and vomiting. More severe nausea and vomiting, as well as severe pain with radiation to the back, may signify complicating pancreatitis. Examination can reproduce the pain, as well as help notice signs of icterus and jaundice of the skin. Patients are usually hemodynamically stable, but the presence of hemodynamic instability, fever, or altered mental status may indicate cholangitis.

Diagnosis
The diagnosis can be made when there are elevated liver enzyme levels as well as evidence of biliary ductal obstruction on imaging. Elevations in total and direct bilirubin, aminotransferases, ALP, and gamma-glutamyl transferase levels are almost always present. The absence of elevation of these biomarkers has a high negative predictive value.[14] In the setting of pancreatitis, amylase and lipase may also be elevated. Elevated white blood cell counts, a left shift, and or lactate elevation could be seen in either severe acute pancreatitis or cholangitis.

A variety of imaging modalities can be used for diagnosis. US is the most readily available one to detect extrahepatic biliary ductal dilation although visualization of the distal CBD may be difficult because of overlying bowel gas. CT scan can also be used; however, magnetic resonance cholangiopancreatography (MRCP) is more sensitive in visualizing the biliary tree. Endoscopic ultrasound (EUS) is an invasive but highly sensitive and specific test to diagnose choledocholithiasis; however, it is expensive, associated with risks, and operator-dependent. Although the sensitivity of EUS is higher than that of MRCP, they both have high specificity; therefore, the decision should be based on cost, patient preference, and availability. ERCP can also be used for diagnostic and therapeutic purposes. Intraoperative cholangiogram can be used to diagnose choledocholithiasis when patients are undergoing cholecystectomy for cholecystitis.

Treatment
Based on the American Society for Gastrointestinal Endoscopy (ASGE) guidelines, patients with choledocholithiasis are classified as high risk, intermediate risk, or low risk based on laboratory markers and imaging.[12]

- High risk (>50% probability): serum bilirubin >4 g/dL and dilated CBD on imaging
- Intermediate risk (10%–50% probability): age greater than 55, or abnormal liver biochemistry, or dilated CBD on imaging
- Low risk (<10% probability): age less than 55 years, normal liver biochemistry, and normal CBD on imaging

Low-risk patients should be referred for an elective cholecystectomy if sludge or stones were visualized in the gallbladder on imaging, otherwise, other etiologies for presentation should be investigated. Intermediate-risk patients warrant further evaluation with either EUS or MRCP to either rule out or confirm the diagnosis. High-risk patients should undergo emergent ERCP preoperatively in the setting of acute cholangitis or evidence of ongoing biliary obstruction such as pancreatitis. If there is no evidence of any complications, then patients can either undergo preoperative ERCP followed by an elective cholecystectomy or cholecystectomy with intraoperative CBD exploration.

Treatment for acute cholangitis includes reversing the obstruction, fluids, and antibiotics that provide coverage for enteric organisms. Hospitalization is needed for these cases, and severe cases require intensive care support.

When to Refer

- All patients with suspected or confirmed choledocholithiasis should be referred urgently to gastroenterology for further evaluation and management to prevent complications such as pancreatitis and cholangitis.
- Any patient with concern for acute pancreatitis or cholangitis should be referred for urgent emergency evaluation

Biliary Cysts

Prevalence/incidence

Biliary cysts are cystic dilations that can occur throughout the extrahepatic and/or intrahepatic biliary tree. The Todani classification in **Box 3** divides them into five categories based on their number and location in the biliary tree.[15,16]

The incidence of biliary cysts is estimated to be around 1:100,000 in Western populations and can be ten times higher in Asian populations. They occur more commonly in women with a female-to-male ratio of 3:1.[17,18]

Pathophysiology

Biliary cysts can be congenital or acquired, and the exact pathophysiology is unknown. Congenital cysts are thought to be related to ductal obstruction or distension

---

Box 3
Todani classification of biliary cysts

Type I cysts (50%–85%): fusiform dilation of the CBD

Type II cysts (2%): diverticula arising from any portion of the extrahepatic biliary duct

Type III cysts (1%–5%): cystic dilation of the intraduodenal portion of the CBD. These can be further classified into type IIIA and IIIB.

Type IV cysts (15%–35%): characterized by the presence of multiple cysts. Further subclassified into IVA, which is characterized by the presence of multiple intrahepatic and extrahepatic ductal dilation, and IVB, which is characterized by multiple extrahepatic cysts without an intrahepatic component.

Type V cysts (20%): One or more cystic dilations occurring exclusively in the intrahepatic ducts (a.k.a. Caroli disease)

during embryonic development or in the neonatal period. It has been postulated that they may occur as a result of an abnormal pancreaticobiliary junction, which leads to the reflux of pancreatic juice into the biliary tree and exposing the mucosa to pancreatic enzymes.[19,20] They have been associated with many conditions including familial adenomatous polyposis, biliary atresia, and autosomal recessive and autosomal dominant polycystic kidney diseases among many others.

Clinical presentation

Most cases are diagnosed in the pediatric age group and typically present with a triad of jaundice, abdominal pain, and a palpable abdominal mass. In adults, the diagnosis may be incidental in asymptomatic patients obtaining imaging for other reasons, or they can be symptomatic and present with abdominal pain, nausea, vomiting, fever, or jaundice.[21] Patients may also present with signs and symptoms of complications related to the presence of biliary cysts, which include pancreatitis, cholangitis, cholelithiasis, obstructive jaundice, gastric outlet obstruction, or malignancy.[21]

Diagnosis

The diagnosis of biliary cysts can be challenging at times. Asymptomatic patients are typically diagnosed incidentally when imaging is obtained for other indications. Symptomatic patients, depending on their clinical presentation, can be diagnosed by imaging either directly or after laboratory tests indicate further workup with imaging such as in the case of patients clinically presenting with complications. Laboratory tests may demonstrate elevated lipase/amylase in the setting of pancreatitis or elevated liver enzymes in the setting of cholangitis or biliary obstruction.

A variety of imaging modalities can aid in the diagnosis of biliary cysts. Abdominal US has a sensitivity of up to 97% for most types of biliary cysts and is more readily available.[22] CT is helpful in detecting all types of biliary cysts and has the advantage of being able to screen for the presence of malignancy. The imaging modality of choice is MRCP, which has the advantages of being able to screen for malignancy as well as not exposing the patient to radiation.[23]

ERCP is the gold standard in diagnosing biliary cysts. It can be used to assess biliary obstruction and the presence of stones in the biliary tree and has the advantage of being potentially therapeutic if needed. ERCP may also be helpful in the diagnosis of biliary tree malignancies as tissue/cytology can be obtained during the procedure. EUS can be used to visualize the biliary tree and has the advantage of the ability to sample any fluid/masses within the cyst to rule out malignancy.

Treatment

The management of biliary cysts depends on their type.[24] Due to the high risk of malignancy, patients with cysts of types I, II, or IV will typically be referred for surgical excision. In the absence of malignancy, type III cysts are typically managed with ERCP sphincterotomy or endoscopic resection. Type V cysts are managed conservatively with courses of antibiotics for cholangitis; however, some patients may eventually require a liver transplant.

Biliary cysts are associated with a higher risk of malignancy, including cholangiocarcinoma, gallbladder, and pancreatic adenocarcinoma.[20] Overall, there is up to 30-fold increase of cholangiocarcinoma compared to the general population, with type I and IV cysts carrying the highest risk.[25] The risk of cancer diminishes after surgical management; however, these patients continue to be at a higher risk of developing malignancies of the remaining biliary tree. There are currently no clear guidelines on appropriate follow-up postoperatively or in patients who elect not to undergo surgery, but periodic surveillance imaging is practiced.

When to Refer

- Any patient, whether symptomatic or asymptomatic with biliary ductal dilation on imaging
- Any patient that has been previously diagnosed with biliary ductal dilation, whether managed conservatively or surgically, for surveillance

Gallbladder Polyps

Prevalence/incidence

Gallbladder polyps have an estimated prevalence in adults of 0.3%-12.3%. The presence of polyps is more prevalent in older patients, with risk increasing around 50 years of age. Factors associated with an increased prevalence of gallbladder polyps are unclear. Only 5% of polyps are considered to be "true" gallbladder polyps, meaning that they are malignant or have malignant potential.[26]

Pathophysiology

The most common type of gallbladder polyps are pseudo-polyps or cholesterol polyps, which account for 60% to 90% of all gallbladder polyps. They are not true neoplastic growths, but rather they are cholesterol deposits that form as projections on the inner lumen of the gallbladder wall. They are formed from precipitation of cholesterol or bile salts. The presence of cholesterol polyps may be indicative of pathologic gallbladder disease such as chronic cholecystitis.

Inflammatory polyps account for 5% to 10% of all gallbladder polyps. They are associated with inflammation of the gallbladder mucosa and wall. These types of polyps are associated with repeated episodes of cholecystitis and acute biliary colic. Both pseudo-polyps and inflammatory polyps have no risk of developing gallbladder cancer. These polyps rarely exceed 1 cm in diameter and are often multiple.[27]

Adenomyomatosis is a more common true polyp. It has classically been considered a benign lesion of the fundus of the gallbladder. However, recent findings suggest these lesions do have premalignant potential. Malignant polyps tend to be singular and more than 2 cm in diameter. True adenomatous gallbladder polyps are considered neoplastic; they are rare and often associated with gallstones. They can range in size from 5 mm to 20 mm.[28]

Clinical presentation

Most gallbladder polyps are asymptomatic; therefore, often detected incidentally. Symptoms associated with pseudo-polyps such as a cholesterol, inflammatory, or hyperplastic polyp may exhibit symptoms of chronic cholecystitis. Right-upper abdominal pain, food intolerance, bloating, and nausea may be present. On examinations, positive Murphy signs may be present. There are descriptions of polyps that protrude resulting in the obstruction of the cystic canal or the primary biliary ducts, causing acute cholecystitis or obstructive jaundice, but these are very rare complications.[29] There are also reports of gallbladder polyps causing acalculous cholecystitis or even massive hemobilia.[30]

Patients with larger adenomatous lesions may have more severe and persistent right-upper abdominal pain. Cases of progressive polyps that have deteriorated into a malignancy may present with jaundice because of growth and impingement of the common or hepatic bile duct. There may also be a palpable mass in the right upper abdomen.[31]

There was no difference in presenting symptoms between patients with benign versus malignant polyps. In a large retrospective analysis found to have gallbladder polyps on abdominal US, 64% of these polyps were diagnosed during a workup of an unrelated illness. Twenty-three percent had abdominal symptoms, and 13% had elevated liver function tests.[30]

Diagnosis

Polyps are most often identified on transabdominal US performed for right-upper-quadrant pain. Abdominal US is the best available examination for diagnosing gallbladder polyps, not only because of its accessibility and low cost but also because of its good sensitivity and specificity. Polyps can occur in conjunction with gallstones but are often seen in the absence of stones. Gallstones are usually mobile, and polyps are fixed to the wall of the gallbladder lumen. Polyps in the gallbladder can be seen in the US only when they are over 5 mm in diameter. Most benign polyps are hypodense and smaller than 1 cm in diameter. Singular polyps that have a tissue density and are larger than 1 cm in diameter carry a higher malignant potential.[32] In cases of diagnostic difficulty with an abdominal US, EUS should be performed.[33]

Treatment

Gallbladder polyps that have the appearance of pseudo-polyps or cholesterol polyps, in asymptomatic patients, can be followed up with yearly gallbladder US. These patients have a very low malignant risk. If serial US reveal that the polyp is enlarging or if the patient becomes symptomatic, then cholecystectomy should be recommended. Patients with symptoms of chronic cholecystitis are usually treated with laparoscopic or open cholecystectomy. Polyps that are 1 cm or greater in size should undergo cholecystectomy because of the increased risk of developing gallbladder cancer. Early intervention is preferred because an early gallbladder neoplasm has a much higher rate of cure than a more advanced lesion.[34]

When to Refer

- A thorough surveillance of gallbladder polyps is needed by the primary care physician and surgeon. Yearly US are noninvasive and help physicians monitor for enlargement, which would suggest the need for cholecystectomy. Remember malignancy is curable if caught early enough.

Gallbladder Cancer

Prevalence/incidence

Gallbladder malignancy accounts for 1.2% of all cancer diagnoses worldwide but 1.7% of all cancer deaths. Overall, the incidence in the United States is lower than that around the world. Only 20% of these cases in the United States are diagnosed at an early stage, and median survival for advanced-stage cancer is no more than about a year.

Gallbladder cancer is the only digestive system cancer that is more common among women than among men. One factor behind the disparity is women's tendency to live longer and high estrogen levels.

Other risk factors include

- Gallstones
- Gallbladder polyps
- Biliary cysts
- Obesity
- Carcinogen exposure
- Typhoid

- Helicobacter pylori infection
- Abnormal pancreaticobiliary duct junctions

Genetics also plays a strong role; 25% of gallbladder cases are considered familial, and certain ethnicities, such as Native Americans, are at far higher risk of malignancy because of limited access to health care as well as diet and lifestyle.[35]

Pathophysiology

Gallbladder carcinoma develops through a series of events before converting into invasive malignancy. Any exposure to carcinogens may convert normal gallbladder epithelium to a condition called metaplasia, which subsequently forms dysplasia to carcinoma in situ, and finally proceeding to invasive carcinoma. The multistage pathogenesis of gallbladder carcinoma begins with gallstones giving rise to a condition called chronic cholecystitis, which increases the risk of gallbladder cancer formation. There is an unusual asymmetric thickening of the gallbladder wall with infiltration to surrounding structures in cases of gallbladder cancer.[36] On the other hand, information regarding genetic and molecular alterations in gallbladder cancer is very limited.[37]

Clinical presentation

Gallbladder cancer detection often occurs as an incidental finding on imaging; therefore, patients are often asymptomatic at presentation or describe vague symptoms such as abdominal pain, nausea or vomiting, indigestion, weakness, anorexia, loss of appetite, and weight loss and can present with jaundice, which can easily be confused as cholecystitis. Biliary obstruction by cancer leads to jaundice, clay-colored stools, dark-colored urine, and skin pruritus. Other nonspecific symptoms of malignancy, such as weight loss and general malaise, may also be present. Physical examination may demonstrate jaundice, right-upper-quadrant pain, or Courvoisier sign (nontender palpable gallbladder with jaundice), which is most likely to develop due to chronic progressive malignant obstruction. Symptoms such as hepatomegaly, abdominal palpable mass, ascites, and bowel obstruction may indicate an advanced malignant stage.

Diagnosis

Patients with obstructive jaundice will need a complete blood count, basic chemistry panel, and a liver function test; results may reveal a cholestatic pattern caused by the biliary obstruction. US and CT are usually the initial imaging studies. EUS is considered more accurate than US (76%) and useful in differential diagnosis to detect histologic neoplasia correctly (97%). EUS will provide a valuable tumor-stage description with invasion depth and local lymphadenopathy. CT has limitations in discriminating benign tumors from malignant ones, but MRCP can help assess the disease extent more accurately and help identify any unresectable lesions.[38] Positron emission tomography/CT can be used to diagnose advanced-stage disease.

Treatment

Neoadjuvant therapy often is not an option because of the advanced disease at diagnosis and is not considered a standard of care in resectable cases.[39]

Surgery is the only curative treatment for patients with stage II cancer or less. For gallbladder cancer incidentally found on cholecystectomy pathologic specimens with stage T2 or higher, the recommendation is to return for further exploration and re-resection.[40]

Postoperative chemotherapy should be offered within 8 to 12 weeks. Adjuvant therapy should be offered to patients with a resected pathologic specimen report of T2 or higher, node positive, and margin positive.[41]

Surveillance includes imaging every 6 months for 2 years, if clinically indicated, then annually up to 5 years.[40]

Unresectable locally advanced and metastatic gallbladder cancers are candidates for palliative goals/chemotherapy.

When to Refer

- Once the diagnosis of gallbladder cancer is suspected, referral to a surgeon should be done for resection. Once the diagnosis is confirmed by pathology after the resection, referral to oncology is recommended for discussion of treatment options.

SUMMARY

Disease of the gallbladder are varied, and many require referral to gastroenterologists and hepatobiliary surgeons. Patients presenting with pain in the epigastric and/or right-upper-quadrant region, as well as those with jaundice and or nausea/vomiting, should be evaluated for conditions of the gallbladder. Ultrasonography is the initial imaging test of choice in most cases. Many conditions will require referral to gastroenterologists and/or hepatobiliary surgeons. Some conditions require more urgent evaluation.

CLINICS CARE POINTS

- Patients with symptomatic cholelithiasis usually have recurrent epigastric and/or right-upper-quadrant pain. Laboratory evaluation is usually normal. They should be referred to surgeons for elective cholecystectomy.

- Choledocholithiasis presents with right-upper-quadrant pain, jaundice, and nausea/vomiting. Elevations in total and direct bilirubin, aminotransferases, alkaline phosphatase, and gamma-glutamyl transferase are almost always present.

- Risk classification of choledocholithiasis guides treatment, ranging from elective cholecystectomy to advanced imaging with endoscopic ultrasound/magnetic resonance cholangiopancreatography to emergent intervention with endoscopic retrograde cholangiopancreatography.

- Be aware of red flag indications of complications with cholelithiasis choledocholithiasis including severe pain, refractory pain, refractory nausea/emesis, fever, hemodynamic instability, and altered mental status. These could signify pancreatitis, cholecystitis, or cholangitis, which all warrant emergent evaluation.

- Biliary cysts are usually found in adults incidentally. Classification is divided into five types, which guides further treatment.

- Metabolic syndrome has a close relationship with the development of cholesterol polyps. A majority of gallbladder polyps are asymptomatic and carry a low risk of malignancy. Patients with symptomatic gallbladder polyps or with enlarging polyps should be treated with cholecystectomy.

DISCLOSURE

The authors have nothing to disclose.

REFERENCES

1. Stinton LM, Shaffer EA. Epidemiology of Gallbladder Disease: Cholelithiasis and Cancer. Gut and Liver 2012;(6):172–87.

2. Alemi F, Seiser N, Ayloo S. Gallstone Disease: Cholecystitis, Mirizzi Syndrome, Bouveret Syndrome, Gallstone Ileus. Surg. Clin. North Am 2019;99:231–44.
3. Shabanzadeh, D.M.. Incidence of gallstone disease and complications. Curr Opin Gastroenterol 2018;34:81–9.
4. Di Ciaula A, Wang DQ-H, Portincasa P. An update on the pathogenesis of cholesterol gallstone disease. Curr Opin Gastroenterol 2018;34:71–80.
5. Mallick B, Anand AC. Gallstone Disease in Cirrhosis-Pathogenesis and Management. J. Clin. Exp. Hepatol 2022;12:551–9.
6. Buckman SA, Mazuski JE. Review of the Tokyo Guidelines 2018: Antimicrobial Therapy for Acute Cholangitis and Cholecystitls. JAMA Surg 2019;154:873–4.
7. Wu JM, Lee CY, Wu YM. Emphysematous cholecystitis. Am J Surg 2010;200: e53–4.
8. Lam R, Zakko A, Petrov JC, et al. Gallbladder Disorders: A Comprehensive Review. Disease-a-Month 2021;67:101130.
9. Bali MA, Pezzullo M, Pace E, Morone M. Benign biliary diseases. Eur J Radiol 2017;93:217–28.
10. Rodriguez LE, Santaliz-Ruiz LE, De La Torre-Bisot G, et al. Clinical implications of hepatobiliary scintigraphy and ultrasound in the diagnosis of acute cholecysitis. Int J Surg 2016;35:196–200.
11. Yokoe M, Hata J, Takada T, et al. Tokyo Guidelines 2018: diagnostic criteria and severity grading of acute cholecystitis (with videos). J. Hepatobiliary Pancreat. Sci 2018;25:41–54.
12. Buxbaum JL, Abbas Fehmi SM, Sultan S, et al. ASGE Standards of Practice Committee, ASGE guidelines on the role of endoscopy in the evaluation and management of Choledocholithiasis. Gastrointest Endosc 2019;89(6):1075–105.e15.
13. Tazuma S. Gallstone disease: Epidemiology, pathogenesis, and classification of biliary stones (common bile duct and intrahepatic). Best Pract Res Clin Gastroenterol 2006;20(6):1075–83.
14. Yang MH, Chen TH, Wang SE, et al. Biochemical predictors for absence of common bile duct stones in patients undergoing laparoscopic cholecystectomy. Surg Endosc 2008;22(7):1620–4.
15. Todani T, Watanabe Y, Toki A, et al. Classification of congenital biliary cystic disease: special reference to type Ic and IVA cysts with primary ductal stricture. J Hepatobiliary Pancreat Surg 2003;10(5):340–4.
16. Soares KC, Arnaoutakis DJ, Kamel I, et al. Choledochal cysts: presentation, clinical differentiation, and management. J Am Coll Surg 2014;219(6):1167–80.
17. Singham J, Yoshida EM, Scudamore CH. Choledochal cysts: part 1 of 3: classification and pathogenesis. Can J Surg 2009;52(5):434–40.
18. Jabłońska B. Biliary cysts: etiology, diagnosis and management. World J Gastroenterol 2012;18(35):4801–10.
19. Babbitt DP. Congenital choledochal cysts: new etiological concept based on anomalous relationships of the common bile duct and pancreatic bulb. Ann Radiol 1969;12(3):231–40.
20. Funabikl T, Matsubara T, Miyakawa S, et al. Pancreaticobiliary maljunction and carcinogenesis to biliary and pancreatic malignancy. Langenbeck's Arch Surg 2009;394(1):159–69.
21. Singham J, Yoshida EM, Scudamore CH. Choledochal cysts: part 2 of 3: Diagnosis. Can J Surg 2009;52(6):506–11.
22. Tadokoro H, Takase M. Recent advances in choledochal cysts. Open J Gastroenterol 2012;2:145–54.

23. Lam WW, Lam TP, Saing H, et al. MR cholangiography and CT cholangiography of pediatric patients with choledochal cysts. AJR Am J Roentgenol 1999;173(2): 401–5.
24. Singham J, Yoshida EM, Scudamore CH. Choledochal cysts. Part 3 of 3: management. Can J Surg 2010;53(1):51–6.
25. Søreide K, Søreide JA. Bile duct cyst as precursor to biliary tract cancer. Ann Surg Oncol 2007;14(3):1200–11.
26. McCain RS, Diamond A, Jones C, et al. Current practices and future prospects for the management of gallbladder polyps: A topical review. World J Gastroenterol 2018;24(26):2844–52.
27. Wu T, Sun Z, Jiang Y, et al. Strategy for discriminating cholesterol and premalignancy in polypoid lesions of the gallbladder: a single-centre, retrospective cohort study. ANZ J Surg 2019;89(4):388–92.
28. Sarici IS, Duzgun O. Gallbladder polypoid lesions >15mm as indicators of T1b gallbladder cancer risk. Arab J Gastroenterol 2017;18(3):156–8.
29. Matos AS, Baptista HN, Pinheiro C, et al. Gallbladder polyps: How should they be treated and when? Rev Assoc Med Bras 2010;56:318–21.
30. Gallahan WC, Conway JD. Diagnosis and management of gallbladder polyps. Gastroenterol Clin North Am 2010;39:359–67.
31. Chang KL, Estores DS. Upper Gastrointestinal Conditions: Gallbladder Conditions. FP Essent 2017;458:33–8.
32. Şahiner İT, Dolapçı M. When should gallbladder polyps be treated surgically? Adv Clin Exp Med 2018;27(12):1697–700.
33. Azuma T, Yoshikawa T, Araida T, et al. Differential diagnosis of polypoid lesions of gallbladder by endoscopic ultrasonography. Am J Surg 2001;181:65–70.
34. Xu A, Zhang Y, Hu H, et al. Gallbladder Polypoid-Lesions: What Are They and How Should They be Treated? A Single-Center Experience Based on 1446 Cholecystectomy Patients. J Gastrointest Surg 2017;21(11):1804–12.
35. Rawla P, Sunkara T, Thandra KC, et al. Epidemiology of gallbladder cancer. Clin Ex Hepatol 2019;5(2):93–102.
36. Roa I, Araya JC, Villaseca M, et al. Preneoplastic lesions and gallbladder cancer: an estimate of the period required for progression. Gastroenterology 1996;111: 232–6.
37. Sharma A, Sharma KL, Gupta A, et al. Gallbladder cancer epidemiology, pathogenesis and molecular genetics: Recent update. World J Gastroenterol 2017; 23(22):3978–98.
38. Furlan A, Ferris JV, Hosseinzadeh K, et al. Gallbladder carcinoma update: multimodality imaging evaluation, staging, and treatment options. AJR Am J Roentgenol 2008;191(5):1440–7.
39. Jayaraman S, Jarnagin WR. Management of gallbladder cancer. Gastroenterol Clin North Am 2010;39(2):331–42.
40. Guro H, Kim JW, Choi Y, et al. Multidisciplinary management of intrahepatic cholangiocarcinoma: Current approaches. Surg Oncol 2017;26(2):146–52.
41. Zamani Z, Fatima S. Biliary Tract cancer. Treasure Island (FL): StatPearls [Internet]. StatPearls Publishing; 2021.

Disorders of the Pancreas

Juhee C. McDougal, MD[a], Neal D. Dharmadhikari, MD[a,b],*,
Sofia D. Shaikh, MD[c]

KEYWORDS

- Pancreas • Pancreatitis • Pancreatic cyst • Pancreatic cancer
- Exocrine pancreatic insufficiency

KEY POINTS

- Efforts to determine the etiology of acute pancreatitis should be made to prevent reoccurrence.
- Chronic pancreatitis is diagnosed clinically based on symptoms, risk factors, and imaging findings. Management includes lifestyle modification and use of non-opioid analgesics.
- The surveillance and management of pancreatic cysts depends on the type of lesion, size, interval growth, and presence of high-risk features.
- Screening for pancreatic cancer is recommended in specific patient population.

INTRODUCTION

The pancreas is an essential organ which lies across the posterior abdominal wall between the duodenum and spleen. Owing to its dual exocrine and endocrine function, it plays a vital role in digestion, nutrient metabolism, and glucose homeostasis. Disorders of the pancreas include a broad range of conditions that are often associated with abdominal pain and reduced quality of life. Although pancreatic diseases are often managed by an interdisciplinary team of specialists, most of the patients will present to their primary care doctor for an initial evaluation. The goal of this article is to provide an overview of several common pancreatic pathologies including pancreatitis, pancreatic cysts, and pancreatic cancer (PC) with a focus on clinical presentation as well as initial diagnosis and management in the primary care setting.

ACUTE PANCREATITIS
Incidence and Prevalence

Acute pancreatitis (AP) ranked number one out of all gastrointestinal (GI)-related discharge diagnoses in 2009[1] and number three most common in 2014 with an

[a] Boston University School of Medicine, 801 Massachusetts Avenue 2nd Floor, Boston, MA 02118, USA; [b] Department of Gastroenterology and Hepatology, Boston Medical Center, One Boston Medical Center Pl, Boston, MA 02118, USA; [c] Department of Internal Medicine, Boston Medical Center, One Boston Medical Center Pl, Boston, MA 02118, USA
* Corresponding author.
E-mail address: neal.dharmadhikari@gmail.com

Prim Care Clin Office Pract 50 (2023) 391–409
https://doi.org/10.1016/j.pop.2023.03.005
0095-4543/23/© 2023 Elsevier Inc. All rights reserved.
primarycare.theclinics.com

estimated annual cost of over 2.6 billion dollars to the US health care system.[2] The incidence of AP in the United States is estimated to be 7.12 to 134.90 per 100,000 person years with an on overall 3.67% increase between 1961 and 2016.[3] In 2014, AP accounted for 351,526 emergency room and 279,145 annual inpatient admissions, an 18% and 15% increase since 2006, respectively.[2]

Pathophysiology

AP is a condition characterized by autodigestive injury and inflammation of the pancreas. AP can be broken down into two subgroups: interstitial edematous pancreatitis and necrotizing pancreatitis. Interstitial edematous pancreatitis can be defined by edema and inflammation of the pancreas and usually represents a more mild self-limited disease course.[4] Necrotizing pancreatitis occurs when there is a progression of edema and inflammation to nonviable pancreatic tissue and can be diffuse (>30% of the pancreatic tissue) or focal (>3 cm in size) and sterile or infected.[5]

The severity of AP varies greatly and can be defined based on the presence of organ failure and local or systemic complications (**Table 1**).[6]

Local complications of pancreatitis include the development of peripancreatic fluid collections (<4 weeks), pseudocysts (>4 weeks, walled off), pancreatic and peripancreatic necrosis, and/or walled-off necrosis.[4,5]

Clinical Presentation

AP generally presents with abdominal pain,[4,5] which can be described as

- Epigastric or left upper quadrant abdominal pain
- Acute onset
- Constant
- Severe in intensity
- Radiating to the back, chest, or flank
- Exacerbated by eating, drinking, and lying supine

In addition to abdominal pain, many individuals also experience fever, chills, nausea, and vomiting.[4,5]

Diagnosis

Based on the Revised Atlanta Classification,[6] a diagnosis of AP is defined by the presence of two of three of the following.

1. Characteristic abdominal pain (as outlined above)
2. Biochemical evidence of pancreatitis (serum amylase or lipase >3 times the upper limit of normal)
3. Radiographic evidence of pancreatitis on cross-sectional imaging

Approximately 80% of patients meet diagnostic criteria by symptoms and elevated biomarkers alone.[4] If diagnosis can be established by abdominal pain and elevated biomarkers, abdominal imaging is not usually indicated.[6] If a patient fails to improve within 2 to 3 days as evidenced by persistent pain, fevers, or inability to tolerate oral intake, imaging is recommended to rule out complications.[5]

After a diagnosis of AP is established, attempts to determine the etiology should be made. The most common etiologies of AP are gallstones (21%–33%), alcohol (16%–27%), and hypertriglyceridemia (2%–5%) followed by iatrogenic, hypercalcemia, infection, genetic, autoimmune, medication-related, and structural etiologies.[4] The American College of Gastroenterology (ACG) recommends an abdominal ultrasound

Table 1		
The severity of acute pancreatitis		
Mild	**Moderately Severe**	**Severe**
No organ failure *and* No local or systemic complications	Transient organ failure (<48 h) *and/or* Local or systemic complications	Persistent organ failure (>48 h)

Adapted from Banks PA, Bollen TL, Dervenis C, et al. Classification of acute pancreatitis–2012: revision of the Atlanta classification and definitions by international consensus. Gut. 2013;62(1):102-111.

in all patients with their first episode of AP to assess for gallstone disease.[5] If there is no history of alcohol use or presence of gallstones on abdominal imaging, then a serum triglyceride level should be obtained; a level greater than 1000 mg/dL is suspicious for causing AP.[5] If the initial workup is negative, then testing for genetic etiologies in individuals less than 30 year-old or pancreatic malignancy in individuals more than 40 year-old could be considered.[5]

Treatment

AP should be managed in the inpatient setting. As there is no targeted treatment of AP, treatment focuses on intravenous fluid resuscitation and early nutrition.

Fluid resuscitation

It is generally accepted that intravenous fluid resuscitation is the cornerstone to treatment of AP. Hypovolemia in AP is multifactorial. AP is associated with fluid sequestration secondary to pancreatic and systemic edema which subsequently leads to intravascular fluid depletion.[4] Patients experience additional direct fluid loss through vomiting and indirect losses from reduced oral intake.[4]

Lactated ringers (LR) is the preferred crystalloid for resuscitation.[4,5,7] There are no set standards for fluid resuscitation; however, ACG recommends aggressive fluid resuscitation with 250 to 500 cc/h of isotonic crystalloid for the first 24 to 48 hours.[5] The International Association of Pancreatology and American Pancreatic Association recommend the use LR at 5 to 10 mL/kg/h for initial resuscitation.[7] Surrogates of intravascular repletion such as hemodynamic stability, blood urea nitrogen (BUN), hematocrit, and urine output can be used guide further resuscitation.[4,5] Although aggressive fluid resuscitation is commonly practiced, guidelines and evolving research have suggested that moderate fluid resuscitation may be a better approach.

Nutrition

The AGA recommends early (generally within 24 hours) initiation of oral nutrition as tolerated.[8] It is acceptable to initiate feeds before pain has fully subsided.[4] For individuals unable to tolerate oral feeding, enteral nutrition is strongly recommended over parenteral nutrition.[5,8]

Antibiotic therapy

The routine use of antibiotics for prophylaxis is not recommended for AP even if the case of severe or necrotizing disease.[5,8] Antibiotics should be reserved for patients with suspected infected pancreatic necrosis[7] or other extra-pancreatic infections.[5]

Risk Reduction Strategies

Gallstone pancreatitis

The AGA and ACG recommend cholecystectomy during the index admission for patients with AP secondary to gallstone disease.[5,8] For those with who are unable to obtain cholecystectomy during initial admission due to need for medical optimization or patient preference, among other reasons, it is recommended that cholecystectomy is completed within 2 to 4 weeks.[4] In cases of necrotizing AP, cholecystectomy can be delayed until inflammation subsides in an effort to reduce the risk of infection.[5] endoscopic retrograde cholangiopancreatography (ERCP) with sphincterotomy can be considered for individuals who are poor surgical candidates or who require a delayed cholecystectomy.[4]

Alcohol-related pancreatitis

Counseling on alcohol cessation is recommended for all patients with AP during initial hospitalization and outpatient.[4,8] Counseling on alcohol cessation outpatient for 6 months in addition to counseling at the time of discharge for AP has been found to reduce the occurrence of AP.[9] Moreover, a Cochrane review article found that brief counseling on alcohol cessation in the primary care setting leads to reductions in alcohol consumption.[10]

Hypertriglyceridemia-related pancreatitis

Patients should be initiated on pharmacologic therapies to lower triglyceride levels to with fibrate and other adjunctive treatments, such as omega-3 fatty acids.[4] Individuals who are overweight should be counseled on dietary and lifestyle modification.[4] In addition, all patients with hypertriglyceridemia should undergo a workup for primary hyperparathyroidism.[4]

When to Refer to Emergency Department (ED)

- Presentation to the emergency room should be recommended for all patients when AP is suspected.
- Refer to GI for consideration of ERCP if choledocholithiasis is confirmed or strongly suspected in patients with gallstone pancreatitis.
- Refer to GI for consideration of ERCP with sphincterotomy in patients with gallstone pancreatitis who are not candidates for early cholecystectomy.

Clinics Care Points

- Characterized by autodigestive injury and inflammation of the pancreas
- Diagnosed based on two of three of the following: characteristic abdominal pain, amylase or lipase >3× the upper limit of normal, or radiographic findings
- The most common etiologies are gallstones and alcohol.
- Treatment with intravenous (IV) fluid resuscitation and early initiation of oral nutrition
- The routine use of antibiotics is not recommended.

CHRONIC PANCREATITIS
Pathophysiology

Chronic pancreatitis is an inflammatory disease characterized by progressive fibrosis and destruction of the pancreatic gland that leads to irreversible exocrine and endocrine gland dysfunction. Chronic pancreatitis can be subdivided into three groups including chronic calcifying pancreatitis, chronic obstructive pancreatitis, and steroid-responsive pancreatitis.[11] Chronic calcifying pancreatitis most often occurs in patients with toxin exposures (alcohol, smoking). Chronic obstructive pancreatitis occurs when there is injury or obstruction to the pancreatic duct, often in the setting of gallstones, tumors, or stricture formation. Steroid-responsive pancreatitis refers to forms of autoimmune pancreatitis which respond well to treatment with steroids[11] (Table 2).

Table 2 Types of chronic pancreatitis	
Subgroup	**Characteristics**
Chronic calcifying pancreatitis	Clinical history of acute pancreatitis with subsequent destruction and calcification of the pancreas Associated with toxin exposures (alcohol, smoking), but can also be genetic or idiopathic Most common subgroup
Chronic obstructive pancreatitis	Obstruction secondary to gallstones, tumor or direct injury to the pancreatic duct causing stricture formation (iatrogenic, post-necrotizing acute pancreatitis, or trauma). Often asymptomatic Rarely involves calcification of the pancreas
Steroid-responsive pancreatitis	Chronic autoimmune pancreatitis Type 1 (immunoglobulin G4 [IgG4]-related) and Type 2 (idiopathic) Often asymptomatic, pain often resolves quickly with treatment Characterized by a rapid response to corticosteroids Rarely involves calcification of the pancreas

Adapted from Majumder S, Chari ST. Chronic pancreatitis. Lancet. 2016;387(10031):1957-1966.

Incidence and Prevalence

Chronic pancreatitis is a relatively rare disease, with the overall prevalence of 25.4 to 98.7 per 100,000 adults.[12,13] The incidence of chronic pancreatitis has been estimated to be 4.35 to 12.6 per 100,000 person years[14,15] About 56% to 65% of patients with chronic pancreatitis are men, and the median age of diagnosis is 55.9 to 58 year old.[14,15]

The two most common risk factors for the development of chronic pancreatitis are alcohol consumption (40%–70%) and tobacco use (60%).[16] Approximately 10% of individuals with one prior episode of AP and 36% of individuals with recurrent AP will progress to chronic pancreatitis.[17] On the other hand, about half of patients diagnosed with chronic pancreatitis do not have a documented history of AP.[18] Therefore, a diagnosis of chronic pancreatitis should be considered in all patients with classic symptoms and/or imaging findings.

Clinical Presentation

The most common symptom of chronic pancreatitis is abdominal pain, which is present in approximately 85% of patients.[11] Of note, the character of pain differs greatly from person to person, with some patients not experiencing any symptoms, but is most often described as.

- Epigastric pain
- Radiation to the back
- Postprandial
- Associated nausea and vomiting

In more advanced disease, patients may experience symptoms of pancreatic exocrine insufficiency (see subsection below) including steatorrhea, weight loss, malnutrition, deficiency of fat-soluble vitamins, and bone disease as well as endocrine insufficiency manifesting as diabetes.[11]

Diagnosis

Chronic pancreatitis is a clinical diagnosis based on the presence of characteristic symptoms, risk factors, and imaging. The first step to diagnosis requires a detailed history and physical. History should include an evaluation of presenting symptoms, prior episodes of AP, risk factors for the development of pancreatitis, comorbid conditions including diabetes, pancreatic insufficiency, bone disease, and family history of pancreatic disease.[19]

If chronic pancreatitis is suspected, potential risk factors should be reviewed in detail to aid in the determination of a potential etiology of the disease (**Box 1**).

Cross-sectional imaging is first line for the diagnosis of chronic pancreatitis. The ACG recommends either computerized tomography (CT) abdomen/pelvis with contrast or magnetic resonance cholangiopancreatography (MRCP) as the appropriate modality.[19] Imaging findings suggestive of chronic pancreatitis include pancreatic calcification, ductal changes (dilation, strictures, irregularity, abnormal side branches), and changes to the parenchymal architecture (atrophy).[22]

When there is a high clinical suspicion for chronic pancreatitis and outpatient workup has ruled out other etiologies of abdominal pain, it would be reasonable to obtain cross-sectional imaging to aid in the diagnosis and expedite workup of chronic pancreatitis pending GI evaluation.

When imaging findings are inconclusive and there remains high clinical suspicion for chronic pancreatitis in a patient, a referral to GI for endoscopic ultrasound (EUS) with or without biopsy and secretin-enhanced MRCP can be considered.[19]

Laboratory testing Is not routinely included in the workup of chronic pancreatitis. Although pancreatic function tests are crucial in the diagnosis of exocrine pancreatic

---

Box 1
Etiologies of acute pancreatitis

Idiopathic	
Toxic-Metabolic	Alcohol
	Tobacco
	Hypercalcemia
	Hyperparathyroidism
	Chronic renal Failure
	Diet (high fat and protein)
	Hyperlipidemia
	Medications
	Toxins
AutoimmuneGenetic	Sjogren's disease
	Inflammatory bowel disease
	Primary sclerosing cholangitis
	Primary sclerosing cholangitis
	Hereditary pancreatitis and Familial Pancreatitis
	Mutations (PRSS1, CFTR, SPINK1, trypsin)
	Alpha 1 antitrypsin deficiency
Recurrent	Post-necrotic
	Recurrent acute pancreatitis
	Ischemic/Vascular
Obstructive	Congenital (Pancreas divisum, Annular pancreas)
	Pancreatic duct obstruction (tumor)
	Sphincter of Oddi dysfunction
	Trauma-related pancreatic duct injury

Data from Refs.[20,21]

insufficiency, they are only used as an adjunct for assessment of chronic pancreatitis as most of the patients with chronic pancreatitis do not have pancreatic insufficiency due to high pancreatic reserve. Testing for levels of fat-soluble vitamins is reasonable as part of an assessment for disease severity. Fat-soluble vitamin deficiency can be assessed by checking vitamin A, vitamin D, vitamin E, and vitamin K (international normalized ratio [INR] can be used as indirect measurement of vitamin K).[19]

Treatment

Lifestyle modification
The initial treatment of chronic pancreatitls targets lifestyle modification and pain management. Alcohol and smoking cessation should be recommended for all patients with chronic pancreatitis as alcohol and tobacco use have been associated with pain relapse and disease progression.[22]

Pharmacologic approaches
Pain should initially be managed with non-steroidal anti-inflammatory drugs (NSAIDs) or acetaminophen. Tricyclic antidepressants, selective serotonin reuptake inhibitors, gabapentin, and pregabalin can also be used as an adjunct in select patients.[11] Opioids can be considered as a last resort option for patients with refractory pain; however, they are not recommended given the associated risks including tolerance and dependence.[19] In alignment with recommendations by the centers for disease control (CDC), opioids should not be used as first line or routine management for chronic pain.[23]

Despite mixed data based on limited trials, antioxidant supplementation with agents such as selenlum, ascorbic acid, β-carotene, and methionine can be considered for management of pain.[11,19,22] Although the mechanism is not well understood, it has been postulated that antioxidants may reduce oxidative stress and inflammation related to pain secondary to chronic pancreatitis.[19]

Pancreatic enzyme supplementation is not recommended for pain control in the abscess of symptomatic pancreatic insufficiency[19] (Table 3).

Invasive approaches
A celiac plexus block can be considered for treatment of pain on chronic pancreatitis. It typically involves injection of a local anesthetic and steroid in the region of the celiac ganglia. With effects lasting 3 to 6 months, it can be a good option for long-term non-opioid pain control or can be used as an adjunct to an oral pain regimen.[19] Endoscopic

Table 3 Initial pharmacologic options for pain management	
Pain Mechanism	**Treatment Options**
Analgesics	NSAID Acetaminophen Opioids
Central sensitization	Tricyclic antidepressant (TCA)Selective serotonin reuptake inhibitor (SSRI) or Serotonin–norepinephrine reuptake inhibitor (SNRI) Gabapentin or pregabalin
Pancreatic inflammation and oxidative stress	Antioxidants

Data from Refs.[11,19]

and surgical interventions can also be considered when pain is secondary to pancreatic duct obstruction from stones or strictures.[19,22]

Total pancreatectomy with islet autotransplant has been used at specialized centers for controlling refractory painful chronic pancreatitis. The data surround its efficacy are limited, but patients who have exhausted all medical treatment option can be considered. These patients should be evaluated by experts in a multidisciplinary setting.[19]

Surveillance
Although chronic pancreatitis has been associated with increased risk of PC, no causal relationship has been identified. This association can be discussed with patients when counseling them. The ACG does not recommend routine screening for pancreatic malignancy in patients with chronic pancreatitis.[19]

Exocrine and endocrine pancreatic insufficiency
Symptoms such as abdominal pain, steatorrhea, flatulence, malnutrition, weight loss, and osteopenia/osteoporosis in a patient with chronic pancreatitis may raise suspicion for pancreatic insufficiency.[19,24] Similarly, new onset diabetes may be concerning for pancreatic endocrine insufficiency.[19] Exocrine pancreatic insufficiency occurs when the pancreas secretes inadequate levels of pancreatic enzymes to maintain normal digestion and generally occurs approximately 10 to 15 years after the patient develops chronic pancreatitis.[24] Patients with long-standing chronic pancreatitis may also develop endocrine pancreatic insufficiency or Type 3c pancreatogenic diabetes secondary to decreased insulin secretion from the pancreas.[24] Although a diagnosis of pancreatic exocrine insufficiency can be made off of clinical suspicion alone, fecal fat measurement generally through a fecal elastase measurement is the most widely available means of testing.[19] Other workup should be done periodically including screening for diabetes, testing fat-soluble vitamin levels, and bone density.[19] Initial therapy should start with 40,000 to 50,000 USP units of lipase supplementation with each meal.[19]

When to Refer to GI

- High clinical suspicion for chronic pancreatitis with inconclusive imaging
- Pain refractory to lifestyle modification and pharmacologic treatment
- Concern for biliary obstruction
- Concern for pancreatic insufficiency
- Concern for recurrent AP

Clinics Care Points

- Inflammatory condition characterized by progressive fibrosis and destruction of the pancreas
- Diagnosed clinically based on symptoms, risk factors, and imaging findings
- Common risk factors are alcohol and tobacco use.
- First-line treatment with lifestyle modification with alcohol and smoking cessation and pain management with non-opioid analgesics

PANCREATIC CYSTS
Pathophysiology

Pancreatic cysts are fluid-filled lesions of the pancreas that are often incidentally identified on imaging. There are several types of pancreatic cystic lesions which broadly can be divided by non-mucinous versus mucinous or by their malignant potential **(Table 4)**.[25,26]

Table 4
Types of pancreatic cystic lesions and malignant potential

Name	Description	Imaging Findings	Malignant Potential	Surveillance Recommended
Non-mucinous				
Simple cyst	Rare in adults	Unilocular, single epithelial layer	None	No
Pseudocysts	Associated with acute and chronic pancreatitis	Encapsulated, lined by granulation tissue	None	No
Serous cystadenocarcinoma (SCA)	Women > men Presents in 50s	Honeycomb appearance (multiple small cysts) with central scar	0.1%	No
Mucinous				
Intraductal papillary mucinous neoplasms (IPMNs)	Most common pancreatic cyst Can cause acute pancreatitis	Direct communication with ductal system • Branch-duct IPMN • Main-duct IPMN • Mixed IPMN	12%–47% 38%–68% 38%–68%	Yes
Mucinous cystic neoplasms (MCNs)	Women > men Middle age Body or tail	Do not communicate with ductal system Ovarian-type stroma	0%–34%	Yes
Solid pseudopapillary neoplasms (SPN)	Women > men Presents 20–50 year old Aggressive	Large, mixed solid, and cystic components	10%–15%	Yes

Data from Refs. [25,26]

Incidence and Prevalence

Estimates of the prevalence of pancreatic cysts vary considerably with one large-scale meta-analysis of asymptomatic individuals undergoing abdominal imaging finding a pooled prevalence of incidentally diagnosed pancreatic cystic lesions to be 8%.[27] The prevalence of pancreatic cysts in individuals younger than 40 year old is approximately 0.5% compared with 19% in individuals 70 to 79 year old and 30% in individuals 80 to 89 year old.[28]

Overall, the prevalence of pancreatic cysts greater than 2 cm in diameter, which are thought to confer a higher risk of malignant transformation, is approximately 0.8%.[29] An estimated 0.25% of cysts are malignant at the time of initial discovery on imaging with an estimated malignant transformation rate of 0.24% per year.[29] There is also evidence that approximately 15% of pancreatic cysts that are surgically resected are malignant.[29] There remains debate on the appropriate surveillance and management of pancreatic cysts given the overall low, albeit measurable risk of malignant transformation, high cost and unproven benefit of surveillance, and high risk of surgical intervention.[25]

Clinical Presentation

The vast majority of pancreatic cysts are asymptomatic.[25] Symptomatic pancreatic cysts may present with nonspecific symptoms such as.

- Abdominal pain
- Weight loss
- Pancreatitis
- Jaundice
- Back pain
- Palpable mass
- Postprandial fullness[25]

Diagnosis

Pancreatic cysts are often incidentally identified on cross-sectional imaging of the abdomen. MRI or MRCP is the preferred imaging modalities for characterizing pancreatic cysts as they are noninvasive, minimize exposure to radiation, and are able to delineate if there is any communication between the main pancreatic duct and the cyst.[25,30] For patients unable to tolerate MRI, CT pancreatic protocol, or EUS can be used as alternatives.[25] Although the above imaging modalities can be helpful in further characterizing a pancreatic cyst, they have overall low diagnostic accuracy and results should be used with caution.

Certain high-risk symptoms and cyst features should raise clinical suspicion for malignancy and prompt urgent evaluation by a gastroenterologist and often a multidisciplinary surgical team (**Table 5**).[25,26,30]

If diagnosis based off of imaging alone is indeterminate and would alter management, then EUS with fine-needle aspiration (FNA) and cyst fluid analysis should be considered.[25] In patients with high-risk features (as above), EUS with FNA and cyst fluid analysis versus short-interval monitoring with MRI should be considered.[25] Cyst fluid analysis generally includes a measurement of carcinoembryonic antigen (CEA) (elevated in intraductal papillary mucinous neoplasms [IPMNs] and mucinous cystic neoplasms [MCNs]), amylase (high in pseudocysts or side-branched IPMNs), molecular markers, and cytology.[25]

Table 5		
High-risk features of pancreatic cysts		
Clinical Findings	**Laboratory Findings**	**Imaging Findings**
Obstructive jaundice without alternative etiology	Elevated CA-19 without alternative etiology	Cyst size >3 cm
		Rapid cyst growth (≥3 mm/ y or >5 mm/2 y)
Acute pancreatitis without alternative etiology		Main pancreatic duct dilation (diameter >5 mm)
New or rapidly progressive diabetes mellitus		Solid components or mural nodule within the cyst or pancreas
Lymphadenopathy		

Data from Refs.[25,26,30]

Surveillance

Most of the pancreatic cysts, even those with high-risk features, are monitored with interval imaging instead of definitive surgical treatment, making surveillance the cornerstone of management.[25]

In asymptomatic patients, the decision to monitor with routine surveillance should consider the individual's risk of malignant transformation, comorbid conditions, life expectancy, and surgical candidacy.[25]

The decision to continue surveillance is a dynamic one and should be reassessed over time based on the individual characteristics. The ACG recommends continued surveillance until age 75, consideration of surveillance for individuals aged 76 to 85 years based on a risk–benefit discussion, and cessation of surveillance if an individual is no longer a surgical candidate.[25] Surgical pancreatic cyst excision is associated with high morbidity and mortality.[25] There is also evidence that medically complex patients with multiple comorbidities are more likely to die from etiologies unrelated to their pancreatic lesion.[25]

If the decision is made to monitor with routine surveillance, MRCP is generally the preferred modality with EUS as an option for those who cannot obtain an MRCP.[25] There are no generally accepted consensus guidelines for surveillance of pancreatic cysts and current guidelines vary slightly from organization to organization.

Pseudocyst or serous cystadenocarcinoma. Pancreatic cysts in asymptomatic patients that are presumed non-neoplastic (pseudocysts) or have characteristic imaging findings of an SCA do not require further evaluation or surveillance unless symptoms develop.[25]

Intraductal papillary mucinous neoplasm or mucinous cystic neoplasm. Screening recommendations for presumed IPMNs and MCNs differs based on the presence of symptoms or high-risk features. For asymptomatic patients with do not have any high-risk features, surveillance is based on the lesion size. Several medical societies have published guideline on the surveillance of pancreatic cyst. The guidelines used in practice in the United States most often are the International Consensus Fukuoka Guidelines, the ACG Clinical Guidelines, and the American Gastroenterological Association (AGA) Guidelines (**Table 6**).[30] Although awaiting a referral to gastroenterology, a primary care provider could consider starting with the most conservative guidelines for early surveillance.

For lesions stable in size and appearance, it is reasonable to extend the surveillance interval, but this can be discussed with a gastroenterologist. For any lesion that

Table 6
Societal guidelines for screening for presumed intraductal papillary mucinous neoplasms and mucinous cystic neoplasms that remain stable

Size	Fukuoka Guidelines 2017		ACG 2018		AGA 2015	
	Imaging	Surveillance	Imaging	Surveillance	Imaging	Surveillance
<1 cm	CT/MRI	• 6 mo • Then every 2 y	MRI	• Every 2 y × 4 y • Then lengthen interval	MRI	• All cysts < 3 cm undergo MRI in 1 y • Then every 2 y for total 5 y
1–2 cm	CT/MRI	• 6 mo × 1 y • Then yearly × 2 y • Then lengthen up to every 2 y	MRI	• Every 1 y × 3 y • Then every 2 y × 4 y • Then lengthen interval		
2–3 cm	EUS and MRI	• EUS in 3–6 mo • Then lengthen interval and alternate EUS and MRI	MRI or EUS	• Every 6–12 mo × 3 y • Then every 1 y × 4 y • Then lengthen interval		
>3 cm	EUS and MRI	• Alternate MRI and EUS every 3–6 mo • Consider surgery in young patients	MRI or EUS	• Refer to expert • Alternate MRI and EUS every 6 mo × 3 y • Then alternate MRI and EUS every 1 y × 4 y • Then lengthen interval		

Data from Tanaka M, Fernández-Del Castillo C, Kamisawa T, et al. Revisions of international consensus Fukuoka guidelines for the management of IPMN of the pancreas. Pancreatology. 2017;17(5):738-753.

changes in size or appearance, there should be closer monitoring with shorted surveillance interval versus EUS with FNA. All patients with high-risk features (as above) should undergo EUS with FNA, if a definitive diagnosis will change management.[25]

All patients with evidence of high-grade dysplasia or malignancy on cytology or evidence of obstructive jaundice should be promptly referred to a multidisciplinary pancreatic center.[25] Referral should also be considered for any lesions that change in size or appearance or that have high-risk features.[25]

Solid pseudopapillary neoplasms. For patients with solid pseudopapillary neoplasms (SPNs) who underwent surgical resection, annual surveillance for at least 5 years is recommended.[25]

Treatment

IPMNs and MCNs with radiologic or cytology features associated with high-grade dysplasia or malignancy can be treated with surgical excision.[25] Radiologic features that should prompt surgical evaluation include the presence of solid components and dilation of the pancreatic duct.[31] Surgical excision carries high risk with an estimated mortality rate of 2.1% and morbidity rate of 30%.[29] Therefore, determining whether surgical intervention is recommended is a complex decision made by a multidisciplinary team including a surgeon who specializes in pancreatic procedures.[25,31]

Surgical resection is recommended for SPNs that typically occur in young women as these lesions are very aggressive with risk of vascular and lymph node involvement as well as distant metastases.[25]

Palliative procedures such as biliary stent placement in a patient with obstructive jaundice secondary to pancreatic lesion can also be considered.[25]

Alternative treatment methods such as cyst radiofrequency ablation[25] or ablation with ethanol and/or paclitaxel have insufficient data to support them and are not recommended at this time.[25,30]

When to Refer to GI

- Patients with indeterminate imaging who may benefit from EUS with FNA and cyst fluid analysis
- Patients with high-risk symptoms or cyst features based on laboratory or imaging findings should be urgently evaluated by a multidisciplinary team including gastroenterology and surgery.
- To aid in determining long-term surveillance of potentially malignant pancreatic cysts that have no high-risk features and remain stable

Clinics Care Points

- Pancreatic cysts are often an incidental finding in asymptomatic patients on imaging.
- Pseudocysts and serous cystadenocarcinomas do not require surveillance.
- Intraductal papillary mucinous neoplasms (IPMNs) and mucinous cystic neoplasms (MCNs) require surveillance given their malignant potential.
- Magnetic resonance cholangiopancreatography is the recommended surveillance modality.
- Surveillance interval depends on lesion size, interval growth, and presence of high-risk features.
- Decision to continue surveillance should continually be reassessed based on patient characteristic and it should be stopped once patient is no longer a surgical candidate.

- Treatment with surgical excision can be considered in IPMNs and MCNs with features concerning for high-grade dysplasia or malignancy.

PANCREATIC CANCER
Pathophysiology

PC is a group of malignancies associated with a very poor prognosis. Most of the PCs are adenocarcinomas.[24] Pancreatic malignancies develop from pre-neoplastic lesions such as pancreatic intraepithelial lesions or pancreatic cysts (IPMNs and MCNs).[24]

Incidence and Prevalence

PC is the 10th most common malignancy in the United States, accounting for 3.2% of new cancer diagnoses annually.[32] The lifetime risk of developing PC is 1.7%[32]; however, the incidence of PC is increasing rapidly on an international level, with 195,000 new cases in 1990 compared with 448,000 in 2017.[33] An estimated 85% to 90% of PC is sporadic, with 3% to 10% thought to be attributed to hereditary factors and 3% to 5% due to an identifiable inherited genetic syndrome.[34] PC overall has a poor prognosis with a 5-year survival rate of 11.5%.[32] Unfortunately, PC is often diagnosed when advanced stage is present, making treatment options limited.[34]

Clinical Presentation

The early stages of PC are often asymptomatic. If symptoms are present, they are generally vague and nonspecific, often present with advanced stage disease secondary to mass effect.[35]

Common symptoms may include.

- Abdominal pain
- Dyspepsia
- Nausea and vomiting
- Jaundice
- Back pain
- Weight loss
- Depression

In advanced disease, patients may present with symptoms of gastric outlet or bowel obstruction, pancreatic insufficiency, pancreatitis, or venous thrombosis.[35] Up to 20% of patients may have new-onset of diabetes mellitus.[35]

Diagnosis

PC can often be diagnosed based on imaging findings alone. The recommended modality of imaging for diagnosis of a pancreatic malignancy is cross-sectional imaging protocoled to assess the pancreas (MRI or multiphasic CT angiography).[35] EUS can be used for staging as it allows for identification of lymph node involvement or vascular invasion.[35,36] It also allows for FNA as tissue confirmation is helpful in management.[35,36] ERCP can be used if stent placement for biliary decompression is indicated.[35]

Chemical biomarkers are not used for establishing a diagnosis of PC. CA 19-9 has a high sensitivity and specificity for PC in symptomatic patients. It can be used to monitor treatment response, disease progression, and prognosis.[35,36] CEA and CA125 are nonspecific and not routinely used.[35]

Screening

Screening for PC is not recommended for average-risk patients.[34] Screening for PC should be considered in certain high-risk groups of patients, including individuals with a history of familial pancreas cancer and known genetic syndromes or mutations that are associated with an increased risk of PC (**Box 2**).[34,37]

The preferred screening modality usually involves both MRI and endoscopy ultrasound.[34,37]

For most high-risk individuals, screening should start at 50 year old or 10 years before the earliest relative was diagnosed.[34,37] For individuals with certain hereditary predispositions, screening should begin earlier. Patients with Peutz–Jeghers should start screening at 35 years. Patients who are CKDN2A gene mutation carriers or PRSS1 gene mutation carriers with hereditary pancreatitis should start screening at 40 year old.[34,37]

A screening interval of 12 months is generally recommended in the absence of known pancreatic lesions. Identification of a concerning lesion on routine screening or new-onset of diabetes in an individual with previously normal screening should prompt additional diagnostic testing or a shortened screening interval. Urgent EUS evaluation should be considered if indeterminate (within 3–6 months) or high-risk lesion (within 3 months) is identified on imaging.[34]

Any patient considered high-risk should be referred to a screening program at the National Pancreatic Foundation Center for Excellence.[34,37]

It is reasonable to stop screening individuals who are at high risk of dying for a non-pancreas-related disease or who are not candidates for pancreatic surgical resection.[34]

Risk factor reduction

Several nongenetic risk factors have been associated with PC. Individuals considered high risk for PC should be counseled about risk factor reduction in the context of risk of PC. Average-risk individuals would also benefit from generalized counseling (**Table 7**).

Treatment

Tumor resection is considered the only curative treatment of PC.[35,36] Unfortunately, surgical resection has limited efficacy, with a rate post-resection 5-year survival rate of 10% to 25%.[35] Treatment of PC varies based on the stage of disease and ability to resect which is determined by a multidisciplinary team based on the review of imaging.[35] Treatment options for local and minimally invasive disease include resection, preoperative or postoperative chemotherapy, and/or radiation.[35,36] For locally advanced disease, treatment begins with chemotherapy and sometimes radiation

---

Box 2
Individuals at high risk for pancreatic cancer

Familial Pancreas Cancer:
- History of PA in two or more first-degree family members
- No known associated genetic syndrome or mutation associated with PA

Genetic Syndrome or Mutations Associated with Pancreatic Cancer
- Peutz–Jeghers syndrome (STK11/LKB1 gene)
- Hereditary pancreatitis (PRSS1 gene)
- Familial atypical multiple mole melanoma syndrome (CDKN2A gene)
- Lynch syndrome (MLH1, GSH2, MSH6 genes)
- Li-Fraumeni syndrome (TP53 gene)
- Hereditary breast and ovarian cancer (BRCA1 & 2, PALB2 genes)
- Ataxia-telangiectasia syndrome (ATM gene)

Data from Refs.[34–37]

Table 7	
Nongenetic risk factors of pancreatic cancer	
Risk Factor	Relative Risk
Tobacco[36]	2
Diabetes mellitus[35]	
Diagnosed <1 y	5.4
Long-standing diabetes mellitus	1.5
Obesity[36]	1.2–1.5
Red meat intake[36]	1.1–1.5
Heavy alcohol intake[36]	1.1–1.5

Adapted from Ducreux M, Cuhna AS, Caramella C, et al. Cancer of the pancreas: ESMO Clinical Practice Guidelines for diagnosis, treatment and follow-up [published correction appears in Ann Oncol. 2017 Jul 1;28(suppl_4):iv167-iv168]. Ann Oncol. 2015;26 Suppl 5:v56-v68.

with consideration of resection for down-staged disease.[35] Metastatic disease can be treated with chemotherapy and supportive care.[35,36] Supportive care can include pain management, nutrition support, and palliative stent placement for biliary or intestinal obstruction.[36]

When to Refer to GI

- High-risk patients should be referred to a screening program at the National Pancreatic Foundation Center for Excellence.
- Consideration for EUS evaluation if imaging identifies an indeterminate or high-risk lesion
- Patient with biliary or intestinal obstruction who may benefit from palliative stent placement

Clinics Care Points

- Often diagnosed when advanced disease is present.
- Diagnosis based on multiphasic CT angiography (pancreatic protocol)
- Screening not recommended for average-risk patients
- Screening for high-risk patients with MRI or endoscopic ultrasound
- High risk defined as ≥ 2 first-degree relatives or known genetic syndrome or mutation
- Treatment based on resectability of lesion, often requiring surgical resection with chemotherapy and/or radiation and supportive treatment of advanced disease

SUMMARY

The pancreas is a complex organ with both endocrine and exocrine function. AP, which is often triggered by gallstone disease or alcohol use, requires inpatient management for aggressive fluid resuscitation and close monitoring for the development of complications. Chronic pancreatitis is another inflammatory condition of the pancreas, which develops secondary to progressive organ fibrosis and destruction. Although recurrent episodes of AP can lead to chronic pancreatitis, many cases are idiopathic or secondary to lifestyle factors or genetic predispositions. Chronic pancreatitis is characterized by chronic abdominal pain that is often difficult to manage and advance disease can manifest as pancreatic insufficiency. Pancreatic cysts are fluid-filled lesions of the pancreas that have high prevalence and are often incidentally found on imaging in asymptomatic patients. Given their malignant potential, certain pancreatic cysts require routine surveillance as well as fluid sampling and referral to a pancreatic specialty center if high-risk features are present. PC is a gastrointestinal malignancy increasing in prevalence that is often diagnosed in advanced stages of disease and has a poor prognosis overall with limited treatment options available. Overall, diseases of the pancreas are often complex, often requiring comanagement by multidisciplinary team. Improved awareness and initial workup and management of these conditions in the primary care setting may allow for expedited and improved quality of care.

DISCLOSURES

None.

REFERENCES

1. Peery AF, Dellon ES, Lund J, et al. Burden of Gastrointestinal Disease in the United States: 2012 Update. Gastroenterology 2012;143(5):1179.
2. Peery AF, Crockett SD, Murphy CC, et al. Burden and Cost of Gastrointestinal, Liver, and Pancreatic Diseases in the United States: Update 2018. Gastroenterology 2019;156(1):254–72.e11.
3. Iannuzzi JP, King JA, Leong JH, et al. Global Incidence of Acute Pancreatitis Is Increasing Over Time: A Systematic Review and Meta-Analysis. Gastroenterology 2022;162(1):122–34.
4. Mederos MA, Reber HA, Girgis MD. Acute Pancreatitis A Review. JAMA 2021. https://doi.org/10.1001/jama.2020.20317.
5. Tenner S, Baillie J, Dewitt J, et al. American college of gastroenterology guideline: Management of acute pancreatitis. Am J Gastroenterol 2013;108(9):1400–15.
6. Banks PA, Bollen TL, Dervenis C, et al. Classification of acute pancreatitis-2012: revision of the Atlanta classification and definitions by international consensus. Gut 2013. https://doi.org/10.1136/gutjnl-2012-302779.
7. IAP/APA evidence-based guidelines for the management of acute pancreatitis. Pancreatology 2013;13(4):e1–15.
8. Crockett SD, Wani S, Gardner TB, et al. American Gastroenterological Association Institute Guideline on Initial Management of Acute Pancreatitis. Gastroenterology 2018;154(4):1096–101.
9. Nordback I, Pelli H, Lappalainen-Lehto R, et al. The Recurrence of Acute Alcohol-Associated Pancreatitis Can Be Reduced: A Randomized Controlled Trial. Gastroenterology 2009;136(3):848–55.
10. Kaner EFS, Beyer F, Dickinson HO, et al. Effectiveness of brief alcohol interventions in primary care populations. Cochrane Database Syst Rev 2007;(2). https://doi.org/10.1002/14651858.CD004148.PUB3.
11. Majumdor S, Chari ST. Chronic pancreatitis. Lancet 2016;387(10031):1957–66.
12. Sellers ZM, MacIsaac D, Yu H, et al. Nationwide Trends in Acute and Chronic Pancreatitis Among Privately Insured Children and Non-Elderly Adults in the United States, 2007–2014. Gastroenterology 2018;155(2):469.
13. Machicado JD, Dudekula A, Tang G, et al. Period prevalence of chronic pancreatitis diagnosis from 2001-2013 in the commercially insured population of the United States. Pancreatology 2019;19(6):813.

14. Olesen SS, Mortensen LH, Zinck E, et al. Time trends in incidence and prevalence of chronic pancreatitis: A 25-year population-based nationwide study. United European Gastroenterology Journal 2021;9(1):82.

15. Yadav D, Timmons L, Benson JT, et al. Incidence, prevalence, and survival of chronic pancreatitis: a population-based study. Am J Gastroenterol 2011;106(12):2192–9.

16. Beyer G, Habtezion A, Werner J, et al. Chronic pancreatitis. Lancet 2020; 396(10249):499–512.

17. Sankaran SJ, Xiao AY, Wu LM, et al. Frequency of progression from acute to chronic pancreatitis and risk factors: a meta-analysis. Gastroenterology 2015; 149(6):1490–500.e1.

18. Hori Y, Vege SS, Chari ST, et al. Classic chronic pancreatitis is associated with prior acute pancreatitis in only 50% of patients in a large single-institution study. Pancreatology 2019;19(2):224–9.

19. Gardner TB, Adler DG, Forsmark CE, et al. ACG Clinical Guideline: Chronic Pancreatitis. Am J Gastroenterol 2020;115(3).

20. Schneider A, Löhr JM, Singer MV. The M-ANNHEIM classification of chronic pancreatitis: introduction of a unifying classification system based on a review of previous classifications of the disease. J Gastroenterol 2007;42(2):101–19.

21. Whitcomb DC. Pancreatitis: TIGAR-O version 2 Risk/Etiology Checklist with topic reviews, updates, and use primers. Clin Transl Gastroenterol 2019;10(6). https://doi.org/10.14309/CTG.0000000000000027.

22. Singh VK, Yadav D, Garg PK. Diagnosis and Management of Chronic Pancreatitis: A Review. JAMA 2019;322(24):2422–34.

23. Lappin R. CDC Guideline for Prescribing Opioids for Chronic Pain — United States, 2016. MMWR Recomm Rep (Morb Mortal Wkly Rep) 2019;65(4):150–1.

24. Kleeff J, Whitcomb DC, Shimosegawa T, et al. Chronic pancreatitis. Nat Rev Dis Prim 2017;3. https://doi.org/10.1038/NRDP.2017.60.

25. Elta GH, Enestvedt BK, Sauer BG, et al. ACG Clinical Guideline: Diagnosis and Management of Pancreatic Cysts. Am J Gastroenterol 2018;113(4):464–79.

26. Ayoub F, Davis AM, Chapman CG. Pancreatic Cysts—An Overview and Summary of Society Guidelines, 2021. JAMA 2021;325(4):391–2.

27. Zerboni G, Signoretti M, Crippa S, et al. Systematic review and meta-analysis: Prevalence of incidentally detected pancreatic cystic lesions in asymptomatic individuals. Pancreatology 2019;19(1):2–9.

28. Farrell JJ. Prevalence, Diagnosis and Management of Pancreatic Cystic Neoplasms: Current Status and Future Directions. Gut and Liver 2015;9(5):571.

29. Scheiman JM, Hwang JH, Moayyedi P. American Gastroenterological Association Technical Review on the Diagnosis and Management of Asymptomatic Neoplastic Pancreatic Cysts. Gastroenterology 2015;148(4):824–48.e22.

30. Tanaka M, Fernández-del Castillo C, Kamisawa T, et al. Revisions of international consensus Fukuoka guidelines for the management of IPMN of the pancreas. Pancreatology 2017;17(5):738–53.

31. Swaroop Vege S, Ziring B, Jain R, et al. Clinical Guidelines Committee. AGA SECTION American Gastroenterological Association Institute Guideline on the Diagnosis and Management of Asymptomatic Neoplastic Pancreatic Cysts. YGAST 2015;148:819–22.

32. Pancreatic Cancer — Cancer Stat Facts. Available at: https://seer.cancer.gov/statfacts/html/pancreas.html. Accessed July 21, 2022.

33. Pourshams A, Sepanlou SG, Ikuta KS, et al. The global, regional, and national burden of pancreatic cancer and its attributable risk factors in 195 countries and

territories, 1990–2017: a systematic analysis for the Global Burden of Disease Study 2017. The Lancet Gastroenterology & Hepatology 2019;4(12):934–47.

34. Aslanian HR, Lee JH, Canto MI. AGA Clinical Practice Update on Pancreas Cancer Screening in High-Risk Individuals: Expert Review. Gastroenterology 2020; 159(1):358–62.

35. Mizrahi JD, Surana R, Valle JW, et al. Pancreatic cancer. Lancet 2020; 395(10242):2008–20.

36. Ducreux M, Cuhna AS, Caramella C, et al. Cancer of the pancreas: ESMO Clinical Practice Guidelines for diagnosis, treatment and follow-up. Ann Oncol 2015;26: v56–68.

37. Syngal S, Brand RE, Church JM, et al. ACG clinical guideline: Genetic testing and management of hereditary gastrointestinal cancer syndromes. Am J Gastroenterol 2015;110(2):223–62.

Inflammatory Bowel Disease

Lia Pierson Bruner, MD[a],*, Anna Marie White, MD[b],
Siobhan Proksell, MD[c]

KEYWORDS

- Inflammatory bowel disease • Crohn disease • Ulcerative colitis • Chronic diarrhea
- Immunosuppression

KEY POINTS

- Maintain a high degree of suspicion for inflammatory bowel disease (IBD) in patients with characteristic symptoms and consider an appropriate workup through laboratory evaluation and endoscopy with biopsy to achieve an early diagnosis.
- Be cognizant of extraintestinal manifestations, which may present before gastrointestinal symptoms.
- Important preventive care in IBD includes colorectal cancer screening, immunizations, and osteoporosis screening.
- Collaboration with gastroenterology is important for both an accurate diagnosis and development of an individualized treatment plan for longitudinal management.

INTRODUCTION

Inflammatory bowel disease (IBD) consists of a subset of inflammatory diseases involving the small intestine and colon. The primary types are ulcerative colitis (UC) and Crohn disease (CD). These conditions have some overlap in symptoms but represent distinct entities that result from various factors ranging from genetic to environmental to immunologic. Although IBD is typically diagnosed and managed by a gastroenterologist, primary care physicians (PCPs) play a pivotal role in longitudinal care encompassing preventive care and symptom management. Most patients with IBD are diagnosed at a young age and require monitoring and guidance for medical management, potential complications, and health maintenance, which should be achieved through collaboration between the PCP and the gastroenterologist.

[a] Augusta University/University of Georgia Medical Partnership, UGA Health Sciences Campus, Russell Hall, Room 235K, 1425 Prince Avenue, Athens, GA 30602, USA; [b] University of Pittsburgh School of Medicine, UPMC Shadyside Hospital, North Tower, Room 307, 5230 Centre Avenue, Pittsburgh, PA 15232, USA; [c] Division of Digestive Health and Liver Disease, University of Miami, Miller School of Medicine, 1120 Northwest 14th Street, CRB, Room 1184, Miami, FL 33136, USA
* Corresponding author.
E-mail address: lia.bruner@uga.edu

Prim Care Clin Office Pract 50 (2023) 411–427
https://doi.org/10.1016/j.pop.2023.03.009
0095-4543/23/© 2023 Elsevier Inc. All rights reserved.

primarycare.theclinics.com

EPIDEMIOLOGY

There are approximately 3 million people with IBD in the United States, with an equal incidence of UC and CD.[1] Although most people present with symptoms in their 20s and 30s, IBD can also be diagnosed in the elderly. There are many risk factors for the development of IBD, none of which are guaranteed to lead to its development. Some consensus protective factors and risk factors are shown in **Table 1**.[2,3]

PATHOPHYSIOLOGY

CD is characterized by intestinal skip lesions with transmural inflammation that can occur anywhere along the gastrointestinal (GI) tract, whereas UC is characterized by continuous superficial inflammation localized to the colon and rectum. Although UC and CD have different intestinal manifestations, underlying pathophysiology is similar and incompletely understood. IBD involves a complex interplay of genetic and environmental factors as they relate to intestinal barrier function, immune response, and microbial dysbiosis. Although no single gene variant appears to be useful for diagnosis, more than 200 gene loci, mostly involving innate immunity and epithelial barrier regulation, have been associated with IBD. The marked increase in IBD incidence in industrialized countries and immigrants moving from low-incidence to high-incidence areas suggests that environmental factors also contribute. Differences in intestinal microbiota also seem to affect the disease processes in both positive and negative ways.

CLINICAL PRESENTATION

Patients with IBD may present with a variety of symptoms that can differ in UC and CD; however, common symptoms include persistent abdominal pain, diarrhea (with or without blood), fatigue, and weight loss (**Table 2**).[4,5] Symptoms do not necessarily correlate with disease activity. Extraintestinal manifestations (EIM) are relatively common and are similar for UC and CD. EIM can include aphthous stomatitis, iritis, episcleritis, uveitis, arthritis, cardiovascular diseases (CVDs), thromboembolism, erythema nodosum, pyoderma gangrenosum, sacroiliitis, primary sclerosing cholangitis (PSC), and gallstones. These conditions can occur before IBD is diagnosed, so PCPs need to be able to recognize these conditions (**Fig. 1**) and should have a high index of suspicion for IBD in patients with these conditions who have, or go on to develop, GI symptoms. Many EIM, other than PSC, ankylosing spondylitis, and uveitis, parallel the clinical course of IBD, giving a window into intestinal disease activity.[6]

Table 1
Protective factors and risk factors in inflammatory bowel disease

	Protective Factors	Risk Factors
Ulcerative colitis[2]	• Appendectomy before disease development • Plant-based diet	• Smoking cessation • Transition from plant-based to processed diet
Crohn disease[3]	• Breastfeeding • Statin medications • Mediterranean diet	• Smoking • Antibiotics in childhood • Aspirin and NSAID use • Oral contraceptive use • Low-fiber, highly processed diet

Table 2
Clinical presentation of inflammatory bowel disease

	History		Physical Examination
Ulcerative colitis[4]	• Abdominal pain • Bloody diarrhea (with or without mucus)	• Tenesmus • Weight loss • Fatigue	• Abdominal tenderness to palpation • Acute abdomen (guarding, rebound tenderness), abdominal distension, and fever may suggest toxic megacolon, a surgical emergency
Crohn disease[5]	• Varies by disease site/extent • Abdominal pain • Diarrhea (with or without blood)	• Nausea and vomiting • Weight loss • Fatigue	• Abdominal tenderness to palpation • Palpable mass may suggest abscess • Fecaluria and pneumaturia suggest fistula • Perianal disease

DIAGNOSIS

The diagnosis of IBD is based on the overall presentation and diagnostic features found during workup, including endoscopic evaluation with biopsy. Initial workup should include a basic laboratory evaluation as well as stool studies to rule out infection and to assess for inflammation (fecal calprotectin; sensitivity 93%, specificity 96%)[7] (**Table 3**). If there is a high suspicion for IBD, consider adding laboratory tests

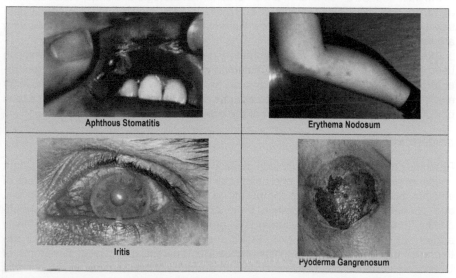

Fig. 1. Extraintestinal manifestations of IBD that PCPs should recognize. (*From* Bouloux P: Self-Assessment Picture Tests: Medicine, Vol. 1. London, Mosby-Wolfe, 1997, p 35, Fig. 69. *(Aphthous Stomatitis)*, and Kühbacher T, Schreiber S. Chapter 9: Approach to the Patient with Inflammatory Bowel Disease. In: Faigel, DO, Cave, DR, eds. 1st ed. Saunders Elsevier; 2008:91-103. *(Erythema Nodosum)*, and Schwartz MH: Textbook of physical diagnosis: history and examination, ed 6, Philadelphia, 2009, Saunders. *(Iritis)*; and *Courtesy* Misha Rosenbach, MD *(Pyoderma Gangrenosum)*.)

Table 3
Initial primary care workup for possible inflammatory bowel disease

Stool Studies	Laboratory Studies	Laboratory Studies to Consider
Stool PCR (or culture)	Complete blood count	Iron panel
Clostridioides difficile (may be included in stool PCR panel)	Complete metabolic panel	Vitamin B12
Ova and parasites	C-reactive protein	Quantiferon gold (tuberculosis screen)
Fecal calprotectin		Hepatitis B (surface antigen, core antibody, and possibly surface antibody depending on vaccination status. Note that this is different from an acute hepatitis panel.)

as needed before starting immunosuppressive therapy, including tuberculosis and hepatitis B testing. Notably, genetic testing and antibody panels are not indicated when making an IBD diagnosis. Given the relatively young age at presentation, the need for endoscopic evaluation, and risks of radiation exposure, computed tomography is usually avoided unless there is concern for an acute abdomen, in which case emergent surgical consultation and imaging may be necessary. If symptoms persist and there is suspicion for IBD, the patient should be referred to gastroenterology to ensure prompt indentification and treatment, thus reducing potential complications.

TREATMENT

In the past decade an expansive armamentarium of biologic and small-molecule therapies has become available to induce and maintain remission in IBD. The general classes of treatment as well as their potential adverse effects and necessary monitoring are listed in **Table 4**.

After an initial diagnosis, anti-inflammatory medication, such as prednisone, may be used as a bridge to steroid-sparing maintenance therapy in consultation with gastroenterology. Surgical intervention may also be necessary depending on the severity and complications of IBD, including strictures and fistulas. This can range from a total colectomy to a segmental resection of the bowel.

COMPLICATIONS

Potential complications of UC include disease recurrence, toxic megacolon, fulminant colitis, perforation, dysplasia, and colorectal cancer. Given the transmural nature of inflammation in CD, additional complications can include stricture, fistula, abscess, and luminal malignancy. In addition, patients with IBD can develop nutritional deficiency, iron deficiency, and vitamin B12 deficiency as a result of disease activity and/or surgical interventions. Both PCPs and gastroenterology should monitor patients for these long-term complications of IBD. Interestingly, clinical symptoms of UC activity correlate poorly with endoscopic evidence of disease severity, so periodic endoscopy is important to prevent undertreatment.[8]

PREGNANCY

Women with IBD can have safe and healthy pregnancies with remission being a goal. Mesalamines, azathioprine, tumor necrosis factor (TNF)-α inhibitors, anti-integrin antibodies, and interleukin-12/23 antagonists do not seem to increase risk of

Table 4
Inflammatory bowel disease medications

Medication Class	Medications (Route)	Mechanism of Action	Pretreatment Testing	Laboratory Monitoring Parameters	Potential Adverse Effects
Aminosalicylates	Mesalamine (oral)	Anti-inflammatory	CBC CMP	CBC CMP (especially renal function)	• Acute interstitial nephritis • Mesalamine hypersensitivity (paradoxical reaction to treatment) • Agranulocytosis with sulfasalazine (rare)
Immunomodulators	Azathioprine/6-mercaptopurine (oral)	Purine metabolism antagonist	CBC CMP TPMT level Consider NUDT15 genotyping	CBC CMP Thiopurine metabolites	• Nausea • Flulike symptoms (fever, joint pain, swelling, rash) • Elevated liver function tests • Low white blood count • Pancreatitis (rare, usually occurs early in treatment)
	Methotrexate (oral or SQ)	Dihydrofolate reductase inhibitor	CBC CMP		• Nausea • Elevated liver function tests

(continued on next page)

Table 4
(continued)

Medication Class	Medications (Route)	Mechanism of Action	Pretreatment Testing	Laboratory Monitoring Parameters	Potential Adverse Effects
Biologics	*Infliximab* (IV) *Adalimumab* (IV) *Golimumab* (IV) *Certolizumab* (IV)	TNF-α inhibitors	• Quantiferon Gold[c] • HBsAb[d] • HBsAg • HBcAb • CBC • CMP	CBC CMP	• URI • Other infections (some serious) • Psoriasis (atypical pattern) • Hepatotoxicity • Fatigue
	Ustekinumab (IV, then SQ) *Risankizumab* (IV, then SQ)	IL-12/IL-23 antagonist IL-23 antagonist	• Quantiferon Gold[c] • HBsAb[d] • HBsAg • HBcAb • CBC • CMP	CBC CMP	• URI • Other infections • PRES with ustekinumab (very rare)
	Vedolizumab (IV; SQ to be approved in the near future)	$\alpha_4\beta_7$ integrin antagonist	• Quantiferon Gold[c] • HBsAb[d] • HBsAg • HBcAb • CBC • CMP	CBC CMP	• Nasopharyngitis • Hepatotoxicity • PML (one reported case in patient with other risk factors)
	Natalizumab[b] (IV)	$\alpha_4\beta_1$ integrin antagonist	• Quantiferon Gold[c] • HBsAb[d] • HBsAg • HBcAb • CBC • CMP • JCV Ab	CBC CMP JCV Ab	• JCV infection • Other infections • Hepatotoxicity
	Tofacitinib[a] (oral)	JAK 1,3 inhibitor	• Quantiferon Gold[c] • HBsAb[d] • HBsAg • HBcAb • Lipid Panel • CBC • CMP	Lipid panel (4–8 wk after initiation, then periodically) CBC CMP	• Infection • Increased lipid levels (not shown to have clinical significance thus far)

Drug	Mechanism	Baseline testing		Monitoring	Side effects
Upadacitinib[a] (oral)	JAK 3 inhibitor	• Quantiferon Gold[c] • HBsAb[d] • HBsAg	• HBcAb • Lipid panel • CBC • CMP	Lipid panel (12 wk after initiation, then periodically) CBC CMP	• Herpes zoster (at higher doses) • Infection • URI • Acne • Increased lipid levels • Hepatotoxicity
Ozanimod[a,b] (oral)	S1P receptor modulator (blocks lymphocyte ability to emerge from lymph nodes)	• Quantiferon Gold[c] • HBsAb[d] • HBsAg • HBcAb • CBC • CMP	• Baseline EKG • Ophthalmic examination • FEV1/FVC if clinically indicated	CBC CMP	• Infection • URI • Hepatotoxicity Rare: • Bradycardia • Macular edema • Decline in respiratory function

Abbreviations: CBC, complete blood count; CMP, complete metabolic panel; EKG, electrocardiogram; FEV1/FVC, forced expiratory volume in 1 second/forced vital capacity; HBcAb, hepatitis B core antibody; HBsAg, hepatitis B surface antigen; IV, intravenous; JAK, Janus kinase; JCV Ab, John Cunningham virus antibody; PML, progressive multifocal leukoencephalopathy; PRES, posterior reversible encephalopathy syndrome; S1P, sphingosine 1 phosphate; SQ, subcutaneous; TPMT, thiopurine S-methyltransferase; URI, upper respiratory infection.

a Approved for ulcerative colitis only.
b Approved for multiple sclerosis.
c Depending on exposure risk, annual tuberculosis testing may be appropriate.
d Consider if vaccination likely done, but no records available.

pregnancy complications.[9] There are minimal data on the small molecules, and some animal models have shown potential fetal harm. Methotrexate should be discontinued at *least* 3 months before conception, and alternatives to methotrexate should be considered in women of child-bearing age. Consultation with Maternal Fetal Medicine can be helpful.

HEALTH MAINTENANCE

IBD independently increases risks for other medical conditions, such as infections, CVD, anxiety, and depression, as well as some cancers.[10] Many patients with IBD are also on immunosuppressive therapies, resulting in further increased risks for certain infections and malignancies. Rates of standard screenings and vaccinations are suboptimal in patients with IBD,[11,12] and intensification of some health maintenance practices is needed to improve outcomes[10,13] (**Table 5**). PCPs and gastroenterologists are sometimes unsure which specific screenings and vaccines are indicated, so systematic education and resources are needed to increase rates.

Disease Prevention and Treatment

Advances in treatment have markedly increased the quality of life of patients with IBD owing to higher rates of symptom resolution and mucosal healing. However, many of these newer immunosuppressive therapies also increase risks for viral and bacterial infections, many of which can be minimized with vaccination. Some of the immunosuppressive therapies, especially corticosteroids and TNF-α inhibitors, can also blunt the immune response to many of the vaccines, including influenza, hepatitis B, human papillomavirus (HPV), herpes zoster (HZ), and pneumococcal, making them less effective. Vaccination before the start of immunosuppressive therapy is preferred, although necessary IBD treatment should not be delayed for vaccinations.

Patients with IBD who are not on immunosuppressive therapy should receive all age-appropriate and condition-specific vaccinations based on Centers for Disease Control and Prevention (CDC) (Advisory Committee on Immunization Practices [ACIP]) guidelines.[14] However, in patients on immunosuppressive therapy, live vaccinations (measles, mumps, and rubella [MMR], varicella, and intranasal influenza) are contraindicated. Patients who are already on immunosuppressive therapy should still receive all recommended non-live vaccines, although immune responses may not be as robust. The rationale for disease prevention and treatment adjustments in persons with IBD is reviewed in later discussion, and specific recommendations are summarized in **Table 5**.

Influenza

Patients with IBD are at higher risk for influenza infections and resultant hospitalizations compared with the general population,[10] making annual vaccination important. These risks are particularly high for patients on corticosteroids. The high-dose trivalent formulation of the influenza vaccine is preferred for those with IBD on immunosuppressive therapy and those ≥65 years old.[13] With increased risk for complications from influenza, patients on immunosuppression also fall into a CDC priority group for antiviral treatment of suspected or confirmed infections.

COVID-19

Patients with IBD with active disease and those on immunosuppression with high-dose corticosteroids and certain medication combinations are at increased risk for severe COVID-19.[15] They should be vaccinated with the COVID-19 primary series as well as boosters based on the CDC recommendations for immunosuppressed persons.

Table 5
Specialized health maintenance for patients with inflammatory bowel disease

Disease prevention and treatment	
Influenza	Give annual high-dose trivalent vaccine for any age on TNF-α inhibitors and those ≥65 y.[13] Give all others annual quadrivalent vaccine. Avoid live attenuated nasal vaccine in immunosuppressed Treat immunosuppressed patients with antiviral therapy for confirmed or suspected influenza infection (≤48 h from symptom onset)
COVID-19	Vaccinate all with primary series and booster doses based on current CDC recommendations for immunosuppressed persons Give immunosuppressed patients early treatment for COVID-19
Hepatitis B	Screen for infection (HBsAg and HBcAb) at diagnosis and before starting TNF-α inhibitors Give complete hepatitis B series if no infection and not previously vaccinated[16] Only if immunosuppressed, check for immunity (HBsAb titer) ≥1 mo after series completion. Further doses indicated if not immune[17]
HPV	Give HPV vaccine series between ages 9 and 26 y. Still strongly consider vaccination between ages 27 and 45 y if not previously vaccinated If immunosuppressed, give 3-dose rather than 2-dose series even if series started before age 15 y
Pneumococcal disease	If no previous PCV13, PCV15, or PCV20 as an adult, give either one dose PCV20 or one dose of PCV15 followed by PPSV23 1 y later. No further pneumococcal vaccines are needed at age 65 y[19] If PCV13 previously received (with or without PPSV23), complete series for immunocompromised patients per ACIP recommendations[14]
Measles, mumps, and rubella (MMR)[13]	Assess for immunity to MMR (receipt of 2 doses of MMR). If no immunization record, check antibody titers If nonimmune, consider 2 doses of live attenuated MMR, with a minimum interval of 4 wk. Hold high-dose steroids and biologics for 3 mo prior and 4 wk after vaccination
Varicella-zoster virus	Assess for immunity to varicella.[a] If criteria not met, check antibody titers[20] If nonimmune, consider 2 doses of live attenuated VAR, with a minimum interval of 4 wk. Hold high-dose steroids and biologics for 3 mo before and 4 wk after vaccination[13]
Herpes zoster	Give 2 doses RZV, with a minimum interval of 4 wk, to all adults with history of varicella infection or receipt of 2 doses VAR[21]

(continued on next page)

Table 5 (continued)	
Follow standard recommendations for other vaccines, including Tdap, meningococcal, and hepatitis A vaccines	
Cancer screenings	
Colorectal cancer	Increase frequency of surveillance/treatment. Refer back to GI if no follow-up in the last year
Cervical cancer (immunosuppressed only)	Follow guidelines for persons living with HIV: annual cytology for 3 y (starting within 1 y of sexual debut), then cytology every 3 y if normal (switch to cytology/HPV cotesting at age 30 y)[25] Colposcopy referral is triggered earlier for atypical squamous cells of undetermined significance with high-risk HPV or any cervical dysplasia (low-grade squamous intraepithelial lesion or higher)
Skin cancer	Visually examine skin annually
Follow other standard cancer screening recommendations, including those for breast, prostate, and lung cancer	
Other screenings	
Cardiovascular disease (CVD) risk	Screen for and aggressively treat CVD risk factors with increased CVD risk Achieve and maintain good control of IBD
Depression	Screen annually and as needed and treat accordingly to improve outcomes
Anxiety	Screen annually and as needed and treat accordingly
Follow other standard screening recommendations, including those for osteoporosis, hepatitis C, and HIV	
Modifiable lifestyle factors	
Smoking cessation	Use evidence-based strategies for smoking cessation counseling to improve outcomes in CD[10]
Diet	Assess for malnutrition/undernutrition, and supplement and/or refer to a dietician if present With limited data, a Mediterranean diet with avoidance of highly processed foods and artificial sweeteners may be reasonable in IBD given additional known health benefits[29,30] Watch for vitamin B12 deficiency as well as iron or folate deficiency with active disease and/or ileal resection
Exercise	Encourage regular physical activity as safe and probably beneficial[31]
Sun protection	Recommend sun-protective practices with increased skin cancer risk
Contraception	Recommend highly efficacious contraception for patients who do not desire pregnancy and are taking medications that may increase neonatal adverse effects

Abbreviations: PCV13 (15 or 20), 13 (15 or 20)-valent pneumococcal conjugate vaccine; PPSV23, 23-valent pneumococcal polysaccharide vaccine; Tdap, tetanus toxoid, reduced diphtheria toxoid, and acellular pertussis; VAR, live attenuated varicella vaccine.

[a] Varicella immunity = Vaccine record of age-appropriate 2-dose series, laboratory confirmation of immunity, or diagnosis or verification of a varicella infection or herpes zoster by a health care provider.

Those with IBD on immunosuppression are also candidates for early COVID-19 treatment. It is important to continue IBD treatment during a COVID-19 infection because discontinuation could precipitate a flare.

Hepatitis B

Reactivation of hepatitis B can have serious consequences, including fulminant liver failure and death. Although it is not clear to what extent reactivation of hepatitis B occurs in patients with IBD on immunosuppression, potential consequences are serious enough that screening for infection is recommended at diagnosis and before starting TNF-α inhibitors. Further workup is needed before therapy for positive screens. Give the complete hepatitis B vaccine series to all patients with IBD who have not been previously vaccinated.[16] For those on immunosuppression at the time of vaccination, the ACIP recommends testing for immunity more than 1 month after series completion (hepatitis B surface antibody, HBsAb) owing to potentially reduced immune response. If HBsAb is less than 10 mIU/mL (nonimmune), a repeat series or a challenge dose followed by recheck for immunity is recommended.[17]

Human papillomavirus

Patients with IBD on immunosuppressive therapy have increased rates of cervical cancer,[18] and HPV vaccination given before exposure to high-risk HPV subtypes is highly effective at preventing cervical cancer and likely other HPV-associated cancers. Three, rather than two, doses of HPV vaccine should be given to patients on immunosuppression even if the series is started before age 15. Although vaccination starting at age 9 and before immunosuppression is ideal, it is recommended for all men and women up to age 26 and is approved for use between the ages of 27 and 45 with shared decision making. Vaccination even in the older age range should be strongly considered, given the increased risks for patients with IBD.

Pneumococcal disease

Patients with IBD are at increased risk of pneumococcal infection before and after diagnosis. Treatment with immunosuppressive therapies, including corticosteroids and TNF-α inhibitors, further increases risk of pneumonia, the infection causing the greatest increase in mortality in patients with IBD.[13] All patients 19 years old or older with underlying conditions like IBD need extra pneumococcal vaccination (see **Table 5**).[14,19]

Measles, mumps, and rubella

With recent measles outbreaks, there has been concern that patients on immunosuppression might be vulnerable to infection. Patients with IBD should be assessed for immunity to MMR, as evidenced by receipt of 2 doses of MMR after 12 months of age.[13] Because of risk of false negative testing, the ACIP does not recommend checking antibody titers in those with IBD on immunosuppression who have previously been immunized. If patients have not been immunized or are tested and found to be nonimmune, the live attenuated MMR vaccination should be considered, but is contraindicated with immunosuppression. Live vaccines should be given at least 4 weeks before starting immunosuppression, or if already on immunosuppression, therapy must be held for at least 3 months before the vaccination and 4 weeks after the vaccination.[13] Delaying or interrupting immunosuppressive treatment to administer live vaccines comes with risks of disease progression with possible emergency department visits, hospitalizations, and surgery, so it should only be done in consultation with gastroenterology.

Varicella-zoster virus
Patients with vaccine records showing an age-appropriate 2-dose series of varicella vaccine, laboratory confirmation of immunity, or diagnosis of a varicella infection or HZ by a health care provider are considered to have evidence of immunity and do not need further vaccination. Patients meeting these criteria should not undergo laboratory screening for immunity because commercial tests have significant false negative rates, especially for vaccine-induced immunity.[13] Patients with IBD not meeting criteria for varicella immunity should have varicella-zoster immunoglobulin G titers checked. If nonimmune, varicella-zoster vaccine should be considered with the same constraints as MMR with regard to live vaccines and immunosuppression.[20]

Herpes zoster
Patients with IBD are at increased risk for HZ even without immunosuppressive therapy. In fact, HZ is the most frequent serious infection in patients with IBD.[13] In addition, patients on immunosuppressive therapy are at higher risk of more severe disease with complications, making prevention by vaccination key. Adults with IBD who have either had varicella or received 2 doses of varicella vaccine are at risk for HZ and should receive recombinant zoster vaccine (RZV), preferably before starting immunosuppressive therapy, and should not wait until age 50.[21] Live attenuated herpes zoster vaccine (ZVL) is no longer recommended, and RZV should be given even if patients previously received ZVL.

Vaccination of household members of patients with inflammatory bowel disease on immunosuppression
Immunocompetent household contacts should be vaccinated with all non-live vaccines to help prevent transmission of diseases to the immunosuppressed family member. Live vaccines can also be given as recommended with a few adjustments. The inactivated influenza vaccine is recommended over the live attenuated version in household contacts owing to the theoretical risk of live-virus transmission. MMR and varicella live attenuated vaccines can be safely given to immunocompetent household contacts, but if a postvaccination rash develops with varicella vaccine, contact with persons who are immunosuppressed should be avoided until the rash resolves.[5] Infants born to mothers on immunosuppressive therapy should not receive live rotavirus vaccine because of relative immunosuppression for up to 6 months from medications crossing the placenta. Similarly, highly immunocompromised persons should ideally avoid contact with stool from infants vaccinated against rotavirus or at least be vigilant about handwashing in the 4 weeks after vaccination.[5]

Cancer Screening

IBD is associated with an overall increased risk of malignancy, with moderate epidemiologic evidence of association with 15 cancer types, GI cancers (including colorectal and mouth to terminal ileum [CD]) as well as extraintestinal cancers (including bile duct and liver, intrahepatic cholangiocarcinoma [in PSC], nonmelanoma skin cancer, kidney [CD], and thyroid).[22] Intestinal inflammation from IBD itself is known to increase risks of GI cancers, and although immunosuppressive therapy for IBD decreases the risk of these cancers, there is some evidence of increased risk of extraintestinal cancers, such as lymphomas, acute myeloid leukemia and myelodysplastic syndromes, urinary tract cancers, skin cancers,[23] and cervical cancer.[18] Patients with IBD should follow the standard screening recommendations for breast, prostate, and lung cancer, but need increased screening for colorectal cancer, cervical cancer (if immunosuppressed), and skin cancer (see **Table 5**).

Colorectal cancer
IBD has long been associated with an increased risk of colorectal cancer, with GI typically directing and performing colorectal dysplasia surveillance. The PCP role in colorectal cancer screening is largely one of coordination to ensure regular GI follow-up, even if disease symptoms are minimal and/or patients are not on immunosuppression.

Cervical cancer
There are data suggesting that cervical cancer screening rates in patients with IBD are not optimal.[18] Although there is no convincing evidence to date that UC or CD by themselves increases the risk of cervical cancer, immunosuppressive IBD treatment does seem to increase the risk of both cervical dysplasia and cervical cancer. Because of this, patients with IBD on immunosuppression should follow the more frequent screening schedule recommended for persons living with HIV.[24,25] Given the increased risks and that oncogenic HPV causes cervical cancer, universal childhood HPV vaccination should be a priority.

Skin cancer
There is an increased risk of skin cancer, including melanomas as well as squamous and basal cell carcinomas, in patients with IBD as compared with the general population.[22] This is thought to be largely, but not entirely, due to immunosuppressive therapy. For the general population, there is insufficient evidence to recommend visual surveillance for skin cancer; however, the risks are higher in the IBD population, and it should be considered.[10]

Other Screenings and Prevention

Patients with IBD should receive all other recommended screenings, including HIV, hepatitis C, and osteoporosis screening. These patients have increased rates of osteoporosis and fractures, but this appears to be explained by confounders, including glucocorticoid use and low body mass index. Given this, patients with IBD should follow the standard recommendations for osteoporosis screening, paying special attention to the indications for early screening based on individual risk factors.[10] Additionally, the screening and treatment of CVD risk, venous thromboembolism (VTE) risk, depression, and anxiety may need to be intensified (see **Table 5**).

Cardiovascular diseases
Patients with IBD have increased risk of CVD when compared with those without IBD, including ischemic heart disease (RR, 1.24), cerebrovascular accidents (OR, 1.18), premature atherosclerotic CVD (OR, 1.27), extremely premature atherosclerotic CVD (OR, 1.61), heart failure (HR, 2.03), and atrial fibrillation (HR, 2.26).[26] These risks are highest during acute IBD flares and corticosteroid use as well as during long periods of disease activity. The mechanisms of increased CVD risk are not completely understood, but may involve a combination of chronic inflammation as well as endothelial dysfunction, dyslipidemia, thrombocytosis, and dysbiosis of gut microbiota.[26] As a result, IBD control is important, as is screening for and aggressively managing CVD risk factors, including calculating atherosclerotic CVD risk and prescribing statins when indicated.

Venous thromboembolism
Patients with IBD are at 2- to 3-fold higher risk of VTE than the general population, with greatest risk with active disease, more extensive disease, hospitalization, IBD-related surgery, pregnancy, and corticosteroid use.[27] Pharmacologic VTE prophylaxis is recommended for patients hospitalized with an IBD flare, even those with hematochezia,

and is safe and effective as long as bleeding is not hemodynamically significant. However, adherence to these guidelines remains low, and education is needed to improve outcomes.[27]

Depression and anxiety

Among patients with IBD, rates of anxiety and depression are high and exceed those in the general population, with overall prepandemic pooled prevalences of 32.1% and 25.2%, respectively.[28] The US Preventive Services Task Force currently recommends that all adolescents and adults be screened for depression, and all persons aged 8 to 64 be screened for anxiety. Appropriate intervals for screening have not been determined, but those at higher risk, including those with IBD, may benefit from more frequent screening. Positive results on screening instruments should be followed up with further assessment for diagnosis and evaluation of comorbid conditions. Patients with depression have worse IBD outcomes, and psychological stress can also worsen disease. Treatment of depression with antidepressants seems to improve psychological and somatic symptoms of IBD and reduce disease activity as well as medical system utilization.[10] Recognition and treatment of anxiety may also be helpful.

Modifiable Lifestyle Factors

PCPs are experienced at counseling patients on modifiable lifestyle changes to improve health. Smoking cessation, diet, exercise, sun protection, and contraceptive counseling warrant additional focus in those with IBD.

Smoking cessation

In addition to the other risks of tobacco use, smoking has been shown to increase the development of CD, speed disease progression, and result in poorer medical and surgical outcomes. Smoking cessation improves outcomes, making counseling and treatment a key focus for those with CD who smoke.[10] In contrast, smoking is actually protective against the development of UC, but given the balance of benefits and risks, patients with UC should still be counseled to stop smoking.

Diet

Some vitamin and nutritional deficiencies can occur owing to active disease and treatment interventions (see **Table 5**). In terms of dietary recommendations, there is little prospective research in the IBD realm. Patients often receive mixed messages regarding dietary modifications, some of which can be extremely difficult to follow. Gluten-free and low FODMAP diets do not appear to be beneficial in IBD without concurrent celiac disease or functional GI symptoms.[29] Data from studies in other immune-mediated inflammatory diseases, such as psoriasis and rheumatoid arthritis, show some benefits with Mediterranean, vegetarian/vegan, and reduced-calorie/fasting diets and might have some applicability in IBD.[29] A randomized controlled trial compared the anti-inflammatory effect of the Mediterranean diet with the specific carbohydrate diet, a commonly used, but complex, therapeutic diet with preliminary evidence of improved symptoms and reduced inflammation in IBD. The study did not demonstrate an advantage for one over the other in CD.[30] With other known health benefits and a wider range of food options, it may be reasonable to recommend a Mediterranean diet.

Exercise

Exercise is safe and probably beneficial for patients with IBD, although recommendations on duration and intensity are not well-defined.[31] Given the increased cardiovascular risk as well as higher rates of anxiety/depression seen in patients with IBD, exercise may be an important strategy to improve health.

Sun protection
With an increased risk of skin cancer in patients with IBD on immunosuppressive therapy, education and adherence to sun-protective practices are important.[10,22]

Contraceptive counseling
It can be empowering to patients to be asked if they plan to become a parent in the next year. For those who do not desire pregnancy, contraceptive counseling is important, especially if they are on medications that may increase risk for neonatal adverse effects.

SUMMARY

CD and UC, both forms of IBD, are seen in approximately 1% of the population and are typically characterized by chronic diarrhea (with or without bleeding), abdominal pain, and weight loss. The diagnosis is based on history, physical examination, laboratory studies, and endoscopic evaluation with biopsy. EIMs may coincide with or precede IBD diagnosis. Pharmacologic treatments have markedly advanced in the past decade, resulting in improved outcomes. Chronic inflammation from IBD as well as treatments that induce immunosuppression increases rates for certain conditions, making collaboration between GI and primary care an integral part of care for the patient with IBD.

CLINICS CARE POINTS

- Abdominal computed tomography scans in the absence of acute abdominal symptoms and inflammatory bowel disease antibody panels are not necessary in the workup of inflammatory bowel disease.

- Follow recommendations for increased vaccinations, screenings, and counseling in patients with inflammatory bowel disease, as completion rates are suboptimal.

- Administer recommended non–live vaccines as soon as possible, but avoid live vaccines in those with immunosuppression, and do not delay inflammatory bowel disease treatment to administer live vaccines.

- Given the increased risk of venous thromboembolism, initiate pharmacologic venous thromboembolism prophylaxis in patients admitted to the hospital with an inflammatory bowel disease flare, even in the presence of bloody diarrhea.

- Encourage regular gastrointestinal follow-up for laboratory and endoscopic monitoring for all patients with inflammatory bowel disease, even those who appear well, as disease activity does not always correlate with clinical symptoms.

DISCLOSURE

Dr L.P. Bruner and Dr A.M. White have nothing to disclose. Dr S. Proksell has given paid educational talks at conferences on inflammatory bowel disease for the Gastrointestinal and Liver Association of the Americas, Baptist Health System Education, and HCP Live.

REFERENCES

1. Xu F, Carlson SA, Liu Y, et al. Prevalence of inflammatory bowel disease among Medicare fee-for-service beneficiaries — United States, 2001–2018. MMWR Morb Mortal Wkly Rep 2021;70:698–701.

2. Kobayashi T, Siegmund B, Le Berre C, et al. Ulcerative colitis. Nat Rev Dis Prim 2020;6(1):74.

3. Roda G, Chien Ng S, Kotze PG, et al. Crohn's disease. Nat Rev Dis Primers 2020; 6(1):22, published correction appears in Nat Rev Dis Prim. 2020 Apr 6;6(1):26] [published correction appears in Nat Rev Dis Primers. 2020 May 20;6(1):42] [published correction appears in Nat Rev Dis Primers. 2020 Jun 19;6(1):51.

4. Rubin DT, Ananthakrishnan AN, Siegel CA, et al. ACG clinical guideline: ulcerative colitis in adults. Am J Gastroenterol 2019;114(3):384–413.

5. Lichtenstein GR, Loftus EV, Isaacs KL, et al. ACG clinical guideline: management of Crohn's disease in adults. Am J Gastroenterol 2018;113(4):481–517, published correction appears in Am J Gastroenterol. 2018 Jul;113(7):1101.

6. Rogler G, Singh A, Kavanaugh A, et al. Extraintestinal manifestations of inflammatory bowel disease: current concepts, treatment, and implications for disease management. Gastroenterology 2021;161(4):1118–32.

7. van Rheenen PF, Van de Vijver E, Fidler V. Faecal calprotectin for screening of patients with suspected inflammatory bowel disease: diagnostic meta-analysis. BMJ 2010;341:c3369.

8. Regueiro M, Rodemann J, Kip KE, et al. Physician assessment of ulcerative colitis activity correlates poorly with endoscopic disease activity. Inflamm Bowel Dis 2011;17(4):1008–14.

9. Mahadaven U, Robinson C, Bernasko N, et al. Inflammatory bowel disease in pregnancy clinical care pathway: a report from the American Gastroenterological Association IBD Parenthood Project Working Group. Gastroenterology 2019; 156(5):1508–24.

10. Farraye FA, Melmed GY, Lichtenstein GR, et al. ACG clinical guideline: preventive care in inflammatory bowel disease. Am J Gastroenterol 2017;112(2):241–58, published correction appears in Am J Gastroenterol. 2017 Jul;112(7):1208.

11. Selby L, Kane S, Wilson J, et al. Receipt of preventive health services by IBD patients is significantly lower than by primary care patients. Inflamm Bowel Dis 2008;14(2):253–8.

12. Xu F, Dahlhamer JM, Terlizzi EP, et al. Receipt of preventive care services among US adults with inflammatory bowel disease, 2015-2016. Dig Dis Sci 2019;64(7): 1798–808.

13. Caldera F, Ley D, Hayney MS, et al. Optimizing Immunization Strategies in Patients with IBD. Inflamm Bowel Dis 2021;27(1):123–33, published correction appears in Inflamm Bowel Dis. 2021 Jan 1;27(1):e9.

14. Murthy N, Wodi AP, McNally V, et al. Advisory committee on immunization practices recommended immunization schedule for adults aged 19 years or older - United States, 2023. MMWR Morb Mortal Wkly Rep 2023;72(6):141–4.

15. Tripathi K, Godoy Brewer G, Thu Nguyen M, et al. COVID-19 and outcomes in patients with inflammatory bowel disease: systematic review and meta-analysis. Inflamm Bowel Dis 2022;28(8):1265–79.

16. Weng MK, Doshani M, Khan MA, et al. Universal hepatitis B vaccination in adults aged 19-59 years: updated recommendations of the advisory committee on immunization practices - United States, 2022. MMWR Morb Mortal Wkly Rep 2022;71(13):477–83.

17. Schillie S, Vellozzi C, Reingold A, et al. Prevention of hepatitis B virus infection in the United States: recommendations of the advisory committee on immunization practices. MMWR Recomm Rep (Morb Mortal Wkly Rep) 2018;67(1):1–31.

18. Allegretti JR, Barnes EL, Cameron A. Are patients with inflammatory bowel disease on chronic immunosuppressive therapy at increased risk of cervical high-

grade dysplasia/cancer? A meta-analysis. Inflamm Bowel Dis 2015;21(5): 1089–97.

19. Kobayashi M, Farrar JL, Gierke R, et al. Use of 15-valent pneumococcal conjugate vaccine and 20-valent pneumococcal conjugate vaccine among U.S. adults: updated recommendations of the Advisory Committee on Immunization Practices - United States, 2022. MMWR Morb Mortal Wkly Rep 2022;71(4): 109–17.

20. Marin M, Güris D, Chaves SS, et al. Advisory committee on immunization practices, Centers for Disease Control and Prevention (CDC). Prevention of varicella: recommendations of the Advisory Committee on Immunization Practices (ACIP). MMWR Recomm Rep (Morb Mortal Wkly Rep) 2007;56(RR-4):1–40.

21. Anderson TC, Masters NB, Guo A, et al. Use of recombinant zoster vaccine in immunocompromised adults aged ≥19 years: recommendations of the advisory committee on immunization practices - United States, 2022. MMWR Morb Mortal Wkly Rep 2022;71(3):80–4.

22. Piovani D, Hassan C, Repici A, et al. Risk of cancer in inflammatory bowel diseases: umbrella review and reanalysis of meta-analyses. Gastroenterology 2022;163(3):671–84.

23. Axelrad JE, Lichtiger S, Yajnik V. Inflammatory bowel disease and cancer: the role of inflammation, immunosuppression, and cancer treatment. World J Gastroenterol 2016;22(20):4794–801.

24. Moscicki AB, Flowers L, Huchko MJ, et al. Guidelines for cervical cancer screening in immunosuppressed women without HIV infection. J Low Genit Tract Dis 2019;23(2):87–101.

25. Perkins RB, Guido RS, Castle PE, et al. 2019 ASCCP risk-based management consensus guidelines for abnormal cervical cancer screening tests and cancer precursors. J Low Genit Tract Dis 2020;24(2):102–31, published correction appears in J Low Genit Tract Dis. 2020 Oct;24(4):427.

26. Chen B, Collen LV, Mowat C, et al. Inflammatory bowel disease and cardiovascular diseases. Am J Med 2022;135(12):1453–60.

27. Cheng K, Faye AS. Venous thromboembolism in inflammatory bowel disease. World J Gastroenterol 2020;26(12):1231–41.

28. Barberio B, Zamani M, Black CJ, et al. Prevalence of symptoms of anxiety and depression in patients with inflammatory bowel disease: a systematic review and meta-analysis. Lancet Gastroenterol Hepatol 2021;6(5):359–70.

29. Jiang Y, Jarr K, Layton C, et al. Therapeutic implications of diet in inflammatory bowel disease and related immune-mediated inflammatory diseases. Nutrients 2021;13(3):890.

30. Lewis JD, Sandler RS, Brotherton C, et al. A randomized trial comparing the specific carbohydrate diet to a Mediterranean diet in adults with Crohn's disease. Gastroenterology 2021;161(3):837–52.e9, published correction appears in Gastroenterology. 2022 Nov;163(5):1473.

31. Engels M, Cross RK, Long MD. Exercise in patients with inflammatory bowel diseases: current perspectives. Clin Exp Gastroenterol 2017;11:1 11.

Functional Gastrointestinal Disorders

Molly Duffy, MD[a],*, Victoria L. Boggiano, MD, MPH[a], Ravindra Ganesh, MBBS, MD[b], Michael Mueller, MD[b]

KEYWORDS

- Functional gastrointestinal disorders • Irritable bowel syndrome
- Functional dyspepsia • Functional abdominal pain

KEY POINTS

- Functional gastrointestinal disorders (FGIDs) including irritable bowel syndrome have negative influences on both the health and lifestyle of affected patients.
- Although causes of FGIDs are unknown, they are thought to be due to abnormal response to antigen presentation, altered gut motility, intestinal mucosal permeability, or alterations in the microbiome.
- Primary care physicians are well equipped to manage most of functional gastrointestinal cases but referral to gastroenterologists is recommended when red flag symptoms are present or for worsening symptoms despite usual medical therapy.

INTRODUCTION

Functional gastrointestinal disorders (FGIDs) are an extremely common set of more than 50 disorders characterized by persistent and recurring gastrointestinal symptoms, such as diarrhea, constipation, abdominal pain, bloating, nausea, and vomiting. Symptoms of FGIDs are heterogeneous and lack structural findings to explain the extent of symptoms. Moreover, FGIDs are common; it has been estimated that up to 43% of adults in the worldwide general population may meet diagnostic criteria for at least 1 FGID at any given time,[1] and they are associated with increased health-care usage and costs,[2,3] decreased quality of life,[4] and decreased workplace productivity.[5]

FGIDs present a significant diagnostic and management challenge for primary care physicians, and represent at least a third of referrals to gastrointestinal (GI) clinics.[6] The pathophysiology of FGIDs remains poorly understood, and diagnosis of functional disorders is made based on clinical criteria with no laboratory or diagnostic testing

[a] Department of Family Medicine, University of North Carolina at Chapel Hill, 590 Manning Drive, Chapel Hill, NC 27514, USA; [b] Division of General Internal Medicine, Mayo Clinic, 200 1st Street Southwest Rochester, MN 55906, USA
* Corresponding author.
E-mail address: molly_duffy@med.unc.edu

Prim Care Clin Office Pract 50 (2023) 429–446
https://doi.org/10.1016/j.pop.2023.03.006
0095-4543/23/© 2023 Elsevier Inc. All rights reserved.

available to confirm a diagnosis. As a result, FGIDs have become associated with significant stigma, including the perception that these conditions are largely psychological.[7] As a result, patients suffering from FGIDs are often less likely to disclose their symptoms to their physicians.[8–11]

Despite these challenges, however, diagnosis and management of FGIDs can often be managed effectively by primary care physicians through engagement in biopsychosocial principles. In this article, we review proposed mechanisms for the development of functional GI disorders, their clinical presentation, initial diagnostic testing, and management strategies.

Prevalence/Incidence

Based on a 2020 survey of adults in the United States, Canada, and the United Kingdom, more than 1 in 4 adults in the general population meet the Rome IV criteria for FGIDs. Prevalence ranged from 4.4% to 4.8% for irritable bowel syndrome (IBS), 7.9% to 8.6% for functional constipation, 3.6% to 5.3% for functional diarrhea, 2.0% to 3.9% for functional bloating or distension, 1.1% to 1.9% for opioid-induced constipation, 7.5% to 10.0% for unspecified FBDs, and 28.6% to 31.7% for any Rome IV FBD. Generally, FGIDs are more common in individuals aged younger than 50 years, and all except functional diarrhea are more common in women.[12] When specifically looking at IBS, this causes a significant burden to health-care systems worldwide. Direct medical costs attributed to IBS in the United States, excluding prescription and over-the-counter medications, are estimated to be as high as US$1.5 to 10 billion per year, primarily due to health-care resource utilization, unnecessary or too frequent testing, and significant regional variation in testing and treatment.[2,3]

Pathophysiology

Although the causes of FGIDs are not always known, there is new research to suggest that in people with predisposed immune systems, antigen presentation to intestinal mucosa may trigger symptoms.[13] A brief overview of suggested pathophysiologic changes is outlined in **Fig. 1**.

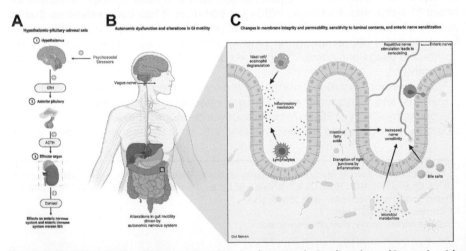

Fig. 1. Pathophysiologic changes occurring in functional GI disorders. (Created with Biorender.com.)

Altered gut motility
Functional dyspepsia, a common FGID, has been associated with several disorders of GI motor function, including rapid gastric emptying, gastroparesis, impaired fundic accommodation, and decreased motility of the antrum and duodenum.[14] This wide array of disorders of GI motor function highlights the heterogeneity of functional dyspepsia, and the need for individualized therapy.

Intestinal mucosal permeability
Studies have suggested a change in epithelial permeability of the intestine, particularly in patients with postinfectious IBS.[15,16] This has been shown to occur via increased spacing between intestinal cells and associated with disruption of the tight junctions between cells, particularly the occludens and zona occludens protein 1,[16,17] which is likely mediated by inflammatory changes driving proteasome activity.[18] As a consequence, there is increased passage of macromolecules from the intestinal lumen to the gut tissue in patients with IBS.[19,20] A similar process occurs in functional dyspepsia with a decreased expression of cell-to-cell adhesion molecules in the duodenum, which compromises mucosal integrity.[21]

Bile acids
Fecal bile acids have been found to be elevated in a subset of patients with irritable bowel syndrome-diarrhea (IBS-D). Bile acids increase colonic transit, which may directly cause diarrhea and increase visceral sensitivity.[22]

Immune-mediated
Biopsy of the intestine of patients with IBS has demonstrated mucosal infiltration of T cells and mast cells in some patients.[23] Further, a subset of patients with IBS (mainly those with postinfectious IBS) did benefit from treatment with mesalazine in randomized placebo-controlled clinical trials,[24,25] suggesting an immune-mediated pathologic condition in these patients. The central role of mucosal mast cell activation is further demonstrated by increased mast cell degranulation and elevated concentrations of mast cell mediators such as proteases and histamine.[23,26] In patients with functional dyspepsia, low-grade duodenal inflammation and increased eosinophil and mast cell presence in the duodenal mucosa were identified, along with alterations in lymphocyte populations in the duodenum.[14]

Visceral hypersensitivity
Immune mediators and products of mast cell degranulation interact with the enteric nervous system to amplify the activation of visceral and somatic pain pathway.[27,28] Additionally, luminal proteases of pancreatic or bacterial origin have been noted to increase colonic sensitivity to distension.[29] Luminal cysteine proteases also have a putative role in the degradation of tight junctions, thereby mediating increased degradation of tight junctions and abdominal pain.[30] Further study has also shown that the local mediators in patients with IBS increase the activation of spinal nociceptors and sensitize nociceptive neurons.[31] Another mechanism that has been implicated etiologically is agonism of the transient receptor potential cation channels, which may be triggered by polyunsaturated fatty acids and inflammatory mediators secreted by peripheral blood mononuclear cells such as tumor necrosis factor and transient receptor potential cation channel, subfamily A, member 1.[32,33] Persistent stimulation of the enteric nervous system in patients with IBS has been associated with an increased nerve growth and density with an increase in mediators of nerve growth such as nerve growth factor and growth-associated protein 43.[34] Increased nerve density may lead to an increased mechanical sensitivity to distension, which

is associated with an increased severity of functional dyspepsia symptoms.[14] Functional dyspepsia has also been associated with an increased chemical sensitivity with an increased symptom burden with acid, lipids, and capsaicin, which lead to an increased neurotransmitter production.

Microbiome

Significant differences have been identified in the microbiome of patients with IBS compared with those without.[35,36] These changes include decreased abundance of *Bifidobacterium*, *Lactobacillus*, and *Faecalibacterium*, with an increased abundance of *Veillonella*, *Ruminococcus*, *Clostridiales*, and *Enterobacteriaceae*. Indeed, transference of this altered gut microbiome into germ-free animals was associated with the development of impairment in intestinal permeability and motility, as well as increased visceral sensitivity in these animals.[37,38] Altered gut microbiome has been proposed to contribute to bacterial fermentation and osmotic overload, which can drive symptoms of IBS. Additionally, there is a proposed contribution of altered fecal microbiota to both alterations in bowel habits and rate of colonic transit.[39]

The altered microbiome in IBS further contributes to the pathologic condition of IBS by the production of short chain fatty acids, which when present in large quantities may activate intestinal T-cells and drive local inflammation.[40] The fermentation profile of fermentable oligosaccharides, disaccharides, monosaccharides, and polyols (FODMAPs) also changes in patients with IBS, again likely secondary to the altered microbiome, with many patients with IBS reporting increases in symptoms when consuming high FODMAP foods.[41] Alterations in the microbiome in patients with IBS also include increases in the population of carbohydrate fermenting bacteria, for example, *Dorea* spp, which are associated with an increased production of gas, which may cause abdominal pain and flatulence, symptoms that are common in IBS.[42]

Similarly, the esophageal, gastric, and duodenal microbiome show evidence of dysbiosis in patients with FD, with these alterations in gut microbiome being similarly implicated in impaired motility and visceral hypersensitivity.

Central nervous system involvement

There is significant overlap between functional neurologic disorders and other chronic pain and psychological conditions including anxiety, and these disorders are often co-morbid.[43] In fact, current thought is that there is a bidirectional relationship between the brain and the enteric nervous system: the brain can exert effects on the GI tract via the HPA axis and the autonomic nervous system, and repeated stimulation of the enteric nervous system and local inflammatory changes in the gut can lead to central nervous system sensitization. The impact of psychological and social stressors on symptoms of functional dyspepsia has been associated with decreased vagal tone, which is associated with delayed gastric emptying[44] along with alterations in brain processing.[45]

Clinical Presentation

Patients with functional GI disorders will present with a range of symptoms including change in stools, bloating, abdominal pain, nausea, vomiting, excess burping or flatus, and sensation of fullness.[46] The symptoms tend to be chronic in nature, often wax and wane, and are sometimes related to food consumption.[47] Symptom severity can also range from mild symptoms that do not interfere with daily life to debilitating symptoms that negatively affect a patient as often as multiple times per week.[47] In some patients, there is coexisting anxiety and/or depression.[47]

Although there is often overlapping of symptoms, clinical presentation is generally dependent on the anatomic location of the FGID. For FGIDs located in the esophagus

Table 1	
Common functional gastrointestinal disorders and associated symptoms	
Condition	**Typical Symptoms at Presentation**
IBS—constipation subtype[49,51]	• At least 25% hard stools • Abdominal pain associated with bowel movements • Bloating
IBS—diarrheal subtype[49,51]	• At least 25% loose stools • Abdominal pain associated with bowel movements • Bloating
IBS—mixed subtype[49,51]	• At least 25% loose stools, at least 25% hard stools, with alternation between the two • Abdominal pain associated with bowel movements • Bloating
Functional dyspepsia[47]	• Fullness • Belching and/or bloating • Epigastric pain and/or burning • Nausea
Functional abdominal pain syndrome[52]	• Constant or nearly constant abdominal pain • Pain is often diffuse and hard to localize to one anatomic location • Ongoing for usually 6 months or more • No clear link to physiologic causes of abdominal pain
Functional bloating[53]	• Recurrent bloating • Sometimes visible abdominal distension • Excessive burping • Excessive flatus

and upper gastrointestinal tract, symptoms include dyspepsia, early satiety, retrosternal chest pain, and sometimes difficulty swallowing. Disorders located in the anorectum might present with symptoms of rectal pain, fecal incontinence, or incomplete defecation. Bowel disorders, the most common of which is IBS, often present with a variety of symptoms including abdominal pain, nausea, vomiting, and bloating, among others.[40]

IBS tends to primarily affect women aged younger than 50 years.[48] Patients will often experience abdominal pain that improves with defecation, and symptoms tend to occur at least once a week for at least 3 months.[48] Patients may have a higher-than-normal predominance of loose stools, hard stools, or a combination of the two.[46,48] They will often have abdominal pain that is relieved with bowel movements, as opposed to some of the other functional bowel disorders such as functional diarrhea where pain is not involved.[49] In more than half of cases, symptoms are often triggered by certain foods.[50] There can sometimes be overlapping clinical features of different FGIDs, which can make diagnosis and management more challenging.[49] **Table 1** below lists some of the most common FGIDs disorders and their typical clinical presentation.

Diagnosis

Diagnosis of FGIDs is based on clinical criteria because no readily available laboratory or diagnostic testing exists to confirm the presence of an FGID. The Rome Foundation has summarized diagnostic criteria for more than 50 separate FGIDs.[54] In general, the primary overarching characteristic of FGIDs is the presence of gastrointestinal symptoms in excess of structural abnormalities or other medical conditions that could reasonably explain the extent of the patient's symptoms.

The most commonly encountered FGIDs in the primary care practice include IBS and functional dyspepsia.[46] Diagnostic criteria for IBS and functional dyspepsia are both contingent on having chronic symptoms that occur on a regular basis and are outlined in **Table 2**.[55]

IBS can be further characterized as constipation-predominant, diarrhea-predominant, mixed, or unspecified; this distinction is contingent on the frequency of stooling pattern by Bristol type, as demonstrated in **Table 3**.[55] Bristol stool types 1 and 2 are considered hard, whereas Bristol stool types 3 to 5 are considered normal, and Bristol stool types 6 and 7 are considered loose

For all patients, medication review should be conducted to identify potential iatrogenic symptom triggers, including the following:

- Antibiotics (eg, trimethoprim/sulfamethoxazole, doxycycline)
- Opiates
- Nonsteroidal anti-inflammatory drugs
- Dopaminergic agents (eg, levodopa/carbidopa)
- Iron
- Metformin and
- Potassium chloride[56]

In addition, a full abdominal examination, including digital rectal examination, light and deep palpation, inguinal lymph node examination,[57] should be conducted. Abdominal examination should include a Carnett sign evaluation to rule out abdominal wall pain.[58] For patients struggling with constipation, complete blood count (CBC), thyroid testing (thyroid stimulating hormone [TSH]), serum potassium, and serum calcium are reasonable first testing steps, whereas CBC, TSH, celiac serologies, and fecal calprotectin can be considered in patients with diarrhea.[46] Combination of Rome diagnostic criteria and a negative fecal calprotectin has a predictive value of nearly 100%.[59] Colonoscopy can be considered, particularly in patients who are aged older than 50 years for whom colon cancer screening would be warranted.

For patients primarily struggling with abdominal bloating or abdominal pain, evaluation with celiac serologies and CBC can be considered. For patients with nausea and vomiting, an initial evaluation may include CBC and electrolyte panel, as well as morning cortisol testing and pregnancy test in appropriate patients. Endoscopy and colonoscopy should be considered primarily in patients with "red flag" indications, such as weight loss, anorexia, age greater than 50 years, early satiety, melena, hematemesis, or family history of malignancy of the digestive system.[46] A summary of the recommended workup based on primary symptom can be found in **Table 4**.

Treatment

Effective treatment of FGIDs considers the role of the gut–brain axis as well as the effects of acute and chronic stress on the pathophysiology and treatment.[60] The first step in the management of these disorders is to provide patient education, reassurance, and to set realistic expectations for the management of a chronic illness. As such, interdisciplinary care and the patient–provider relationship have been shown to improve patient and provider satisfaction, adherence to treatment, and improved clinical outcomes.[51] Given the broad range of presenting symptoms patients may experience and the fluctuation in clinical profile and severity over time, clinicians must identify which of these particular factors are targets for treatment.[46] In addition to discussing overarching themes in the treatment of FGIDs, this section will focus on management of the 4 of the most common diagnoses—IBS-C, IBS-D, functional dyspepsia, and functional abdominal pain.

Table 2
Rome IV diagnostic criteria for irritable bowel syndrome and functional dyspepsia

Condition	Symptom Frequency:	Symptom Duration:	Number of Criteria Needed for Diagnosis:	Criteria:
IBS	1 d/wk	At least 3 mo	>2	1. Pain related to defecation 2. Pain associated with a change in stool frequency 3. Pain associated with a change in stool appearance
Functional dyspepsia	4 times/mo	At least 2 mo	>1	1. Postprandial fullness 2. Early satiety 3. Epigastric pain or burning not associated with defecation 4. Absence of another medical condition to explain symptoms

Psychosocial Treatment

Recent guidelines from the American College of Gastroenterology (ACG) do suggest using gut-directed psychotherapies to treat global IBS symptoms; however, the quality of evidence is very low.[61] These treatments include cognitive behavioral therapy in addition to gut-directed hypnotherapy. Other areas that have been studied include relaxation training, mindfulness meditation training, and stress management. A 2019 systematic review and meta-analysis investigated the effects of psychological therapies in IBS and did find that overall psychological therapies do seem to be effective treatment of IBS. Notably, there were limitations in the quality of the evidence and treatment effects may be overestimated. Self-administered CBT, stress management, mindfulness training, and CBT delivered via the Internet were found to be of no benefit.[62] Despite the lack of quality evidence, given the low risk of behavioral based interventions, referral for gut-directed psychotherapies may be beneficial in patients who are open to behavioral change to alleviate symptoms. Patients who have limited insight into the gut–brain interaction or who are unable or unwilling to commit to treatment are unlikely to benefit from this intervention.[46,61,63]

Lifestyle Modifications

Dietary changes have been shown to improve IBS symptoms, in particular the elimination of FODMAPs and a trial of a low FODMAP diet is recommended in the most recent ACG guidelines.[61,64] Components of a low FODMAP diet are outlined in **Table 5**.

Traditional IBS dietary advice, including a regular meal pattern, avoidance of large meals, and reduced intake of fat, insoluble fibers, caffeine, and gas-producing foods, has also been shown to reduce the severity of IBS symptoms.[65] The data for gluten avoidance are mixed. Some studies suggest that a small proportion of patients with IBS have an intolerance to gluten; however, the benefits of gluten-free or low-gluten diets in patients without celiac disease are limited.[66] As such, it is not routinely suggested for patients with FGIDs to try gluten-free diets; however, a food diary could be considered. ACG clinical guidelines recommend against routine food allergy testing in patients with IBS because this has a low specificity for the detection of true allergies.[61]

Table 3
Diagnostic criteria for irritable bowel syndrome subtypes

IBS Subtype	Proportion of Bristol 1–2 Stools:	Proportion of Bristol 6–7 Stools:
IBS-C	>25%	<25%
IBS-D	<25%	>25%
IBS-M	>25%	>25%
IBS-U	All patients who cannot be classified into the above 3 groups	

Soluble fiber has been shown to improve symptoms in global IBS symptoms, particularly when constipation is the primary symptom. Soluble fiber can be found in psyllium, oat, bran, barley, and beans. In contrast, insoluble fiber has been shown to cause bloating and increased flatulence and should be avoided. This is typically found in wheat bran, whole grains, and some vegetables.[61]

The use of peppermint has been recommended for relief of global IBS symptoms because this is typically well tolerated and has been shown to improve abdominal pain. However, this is contraindicated in patients with GERD because this can affect the lower esophageal sphincter function.[61]

In addition to dietary modifications, increased physical activity has been shown to improve symptoms in IBS. A 2011 randomized controlled trial demonstrated that increased physical activity composed of 20 to 60 minutes of moderate-to-vigorous activity 3 to 5 days per week resulted in decreased severity of IBS, as well as prevention of deterioration of symptoms.[67]

Table 4
Diagnostic considerations by primary symptom for patients suspected of having a functional gastrointestinal disorder

Primary Symptom	Testing Considerations
Nausea Vomiting	CBC with differential Electrolyte panel Pregnancy test Morning cortisol level Upper endoscopy
Abdominal bloating	CBC with differential Celiac serologies
Abdominal pain	CBC with differential Celiac serologies Endoscopy Colonoscopy
Constipation	Potassium Calcium CBC with differential TSH Colonoscopy
Diarrhea	CBC with differential Thyroid stimulating hormone Celiac serologies Fecal calprotectin Colonoscopy

Table 5
Components of a low fermentable oligosaccharides, disaccharides, monosaccharides, and polyol diet and examples of food to avoid

	Compounds	Examples of Foods to Avoid
Fermented		
Oligosaccharides	Fructans and galacto-oligosaccharide	Wheat and rye products Legumes Nuts Artichokes Onions Garlic
Disaccharide	Lactose	Milk products
Monosaccharide	Fructose	Apples Pears Watermelon Mango Honey Commercial sweeteners High fructose corn syrup
And		
Polyols	Mannitol, sorbitol, xylitol, and isomalt	Apples Pears Stone fruits Cauliflower Mushrooms Snow peas Sugar-free chewing gum and mints

Data from Barrett JS. How to institute the low-FODMAP diet. J Gastroenterol Hepatol. 2017;32 Suppl 1:8-10.

Pharmacologic Therapy

In patients with persistent symptoms of FGIDs despite appropriate nonpharmacologic interventions, pharmacologic therapy can be considered. Treatment should be based on the predominant symptom and considered when symptoms are actively affecting quality of life. Given the evolving nature of functional disorders, treatments may need to be altered over time. This section will discuss recommended management of common symptoms including constipation, diarrhea, dyspepsia, and abdominal pain. **Table 6** will review recommended dosing of the listed medications.

Constipation

Initial management of constipation should be attempted with soluble fiber, followed by a trial of polyethylene glycol (PEG). Evidence is somewhat mixed for the use of PEG in IBS because it does not improve abdominal pain or bloating but may be beneficial in patients with primarily constipation.[68] For symptoms refractory to both of these measures, chloride channel activators (lubiprostone) versus guanylate cyclase activators (linaclotide and plecanatide) can be considered. Lubiprostone is approved for women with IBS-C and has been shown to improve abdominal pain and discomfort in addition to stool frequency.[69] Similarly, linaclotide and plecanatide are approved for patients with persistent constipation despite treatment with PEG and have been shown to improve global IBS symptoms.[70] For patients who have persistent symptoms despite the above therapies, tenapanor (NHE3 inhibitor) could be considered because it has

Table 6
Pharmacotherapy in treatment of functional gastrointestinal disorders

Symptom Target	Class of Medication	Dosing	Mechanism of Action	Side Effects
Constipation	Osmotic laxatives	PEG: 17 g dissolved in 8 ounces of water once daily, titrate up or down to maximum of 34 g daily	Induces catharsis by osmotic effects	Flatulence (7%) Nausea (6%) Loose stools (4%)
	Chloride channel activators	Lubiprostone: 8 μg twice daily	Activation of these receptors increases intestinal secretion and peristalsis	Diarrhea (6%–14%) Nausea (8%–19%) can reduce by consuming with meals
	Guanylate cyclase activators	Linaclotide 290 μg Plecanatide 3 mg Discontinue if not responding in 4 wk	Classified as a secretagogue - activates GC-C receptors, increasing intestinal fluid secretion and peristalsis	Diarrhea (16%–22%)
	NHE3 inhibitor	Tenapanor 50 mg bid Discontinue if no response in 4 wk	Sodium hydrogen exchanger, enhances intestinal fluid volume and transit	Diarrhea (15%–16%)
Diarrhea	Antidiarrheal	Loperamide 2 mg 45 min before meals No new data	Inhibits peristalsis and antisecretory activity and prolongs intestinal transit time	Constipation (2%–5%)
	Mixed opioid agonists and antagonists	Eluxadoline 100 mg twice daily 75 mg twice daily can be used in patients with hepatic disease	Mixed mu and kappa opioid receptor agonist and delta opioid receptor antagonist	Constipation (8%) Nausea (7%) Abdominal pain (7%)
	Antibiotics	Rifaximin 550 mg 3 times daily for 14 d, can repeat 2 times with same regimen		Peripheral edema (15%) Nausea (14%) Dizziness (13%)
	5-HT3 antagonist	Alosetron 0.5 mg BID, can increase to 1 mg twice per day, stop if not improving after 4 wk	Modulates visceral afferent activity, decreasing colonic motility and secretion	Constipation (9%–29%)

Dyspepsia	Proton pump inhibitors	Omeprazole 20 mg daily Lansoprazole 30 mg daily Pantoprazole 40 mg daily	Suppresses gastric basal and stimulated acid secretion	Significant long-term effects, recommended trial off every 6–12 mo
	Prokinetic agents	Metoclopramide 5–10 mg 3 times daily 30 min before meals and at night for 4 wk	Causes enhanced motility and accelerated gastric emptying, increases lower esophageal sphincter tone	Drowsiness (10%–70%)
Abdominal pain	TCAs	Amitriptyline, nortriptyline, desipramine, and imipramine—start at 10–25 mg at night, can gradually increase by 25 mg every 4 wk to target dose of 50–100 mg nightly	Increases synaptic concentration of serotonin and norepinephrine, anticholinergic effects may slow GI transit	Not recommended in patients aged older than 65 y
	Antispasmodics	Dicyclomine 10–20 mg 3–4 times daily Hyoscamine IR 0.125–0.25 every 4–8 h as needed, maximum 1.5 mg/d	Blocks acetylcholine at parasympathetic sites in smooth muscle, secretory glands, and the central nervous system	Nausea (14%) Xerostomia (33%) Dizziness (40%) Blurred vision (27%)

been shown to improve global IBS-C symptoms. Previously, tegaserod (5-HT4 receptor agonist) was used in cases of resistant IBS-C; however, as of July 2022, this medication was withdrawn from the market.

Diarrhea

Treatment of IBS-D generally starts with the use of antidiarrheals, particularly loperamide. Data are fairly limited and comes primarily from 2 small RCTs; however, this was shown to be effective in the reduction of diarrhea and is recommended by the American Gastroenterological Association (AGA). Alosetron is approved for IBS-D in female patients whose symptoms have failed to respond to other treatments and may be effective in reducing abdominal pain and diarrhea. Rifaximin in short courses has been shown to be effective in decreasing abdominal pain and bloating. Eluxadoline can be used in patients with severe IBS-D that is refractory to all other agents but has a high association with severe acute pancreatitis and is contraindicated in patients who have a history of biliary disorders, pancreatitis, and heavy alcohol use.[61,71]

Dyspepsia

Specific treatments for functional dyspepsia include a trial of proton pump inhibitors (PPIs). These have been shown to have efficacy in the treatment of dyspepsia and should be used once daily. Unlike PPIs, histamine-2 receptor antagonists have poor evidence to support their use and are not routinely recommended. In patients who do not show an adequate response to PPIs within 8 weeks, tricyclic antidepressants (TCAs) can be considered (discussed below). Finally, prokinetic agents have been shown to have some efficacy in improving symptoms; however, given significant risk of adverse effects, these are limited to 4-week trials.[72,73]

Abdominal Pain

Treatment of functional abdominal pain should first be directed at treating underlying constipation, diarrhea, or dyspepsia. If symptoms do not improve, additional agents can be used to attempt to address abdominal pain. TCAs have the strongest evidence in treating FGIDs and are thought to improve visceral pain and central pain, in addition to slowing GI transit via their anticholinergic effects. In contrast to TCAs, neither selective serotonin reuptake inhibitors nor selective norepinephrine reuptake inhibitors have been shown to have significant benefit in treating IBS, unless the patient has other indications for this class of medications. Data for antispasmodics for patients with IBS are mixed. Current ACG guidelines recommend against use, whereas the AGA suggests that use can be beneficial. Overall, these medications may provide short-term relief in symptoms of abdominal pain but long-term efficacy has not been shown.[61,71]

Treatments to Avoid

A brief list of treatments to avoid in the management of FGIDs are listed in **Table 7**.

When to Refer

Oftentimes, FGIDs can be managed by primary care physicians without the need for referral. In addition, some studies have found that more than one-third of patients referred to outpatient gastroenterology clinics will ultimately be diagnosed with FGIDs, a statistical that has been relatively unchanged since at least the 1980s.[6] Nevertheless, there are certain indications for gastroenterology clinic referral, even for patients with established diagnoses of FGIDs. Symptoms such as melena or worsening dyspepsia despite usual medical care might warrant an endoscopic evaluation. Rectal bleeding and iron deficiency might warrant a colonoscopy. Other referral indications include unexplained elevation in inflammatory markers or new anemia, elevated fecal

Table 7
Treatments with limited evidence in functional gastrointestinal disorders

Modality	Evidence Against
Opiates	Should be avoided in the treatment of functional GI disorders due to lack of evidence of efficacy in addition to concerning side effects, risk of tolerance and habituation, risk of overdose, and risk of withdrawal
Benzodiazepines	Lack of data to support efficacy in functional disorders, may have side effects such as habituation, withdrawal, and drug interactions[74]
Bile acid sequestrants	Not recommended by the ACG due to lack of testing for bile acid malabsorption in addition to lack of controlled trials of bile acid sequestrants inpatients with IBS-D. Side effects also include bloating, flatulence, abdominal discomfort, and constipation[61]
Probiotics	There is some evidence that they may be effective; however, the studies are difficult to interpret given the multiple strains of probiotics and the lack of trials based on FDA endpoints[61,75]
Fecal transplant	It is possible that alterations in the gut microbiome may lead to the development of IBS, so it is hypothesized that fecal transplant could be beneficial; however, there is limited evidence to suggest that this would be efficacious in treatment of IBS. Significant research is needed before this can be recommended[61]

calprotectin, age of presentation older than 50 years, family history of colonic inflammatory processes such as inflammatory bowel disorders (IBDs) or colon cancer, persistent or progressive symptoms despite usual medical care, or weight loss.[76]

Physicians may choose to refer patients to psychologists for therapy at various points in the treatment course. Although patients may assume that there are only biomedical reasons for their functional GI symptoms, therapy services can help to uncover mental health conditions that may be linked to and largely responsible for symptoms.[77] Moreover, given the high link between FGIDs and major depressive disorder or generalized anxiety disorder, a large proportion of patients benefit from coexisting referrals to mental health professionals as early as 3 to 6 months after beginning medical therapy.[77]

SUMMARY

FGIDs include more than 50 conditions along the gastrointestinal tract that present with a variety of symptoms and have significant negative impact on the health and lifestyle of affected patients. The most common FGID is IBS, which includes diarrhea, constipation, mixed, and unclassified subtypes. The economic impact of FGIDs is significant. Direct medical costs for IBS alone range from US$1.5 to 10 billion.[2,3] Although the cause of FGIDs remains largely unknown, possible causal mechanisms include altered gut motility, intestinal mucosal permeability, alterations in patients' microbiome, bile acid elevation, or immune activation after antigen presentation to intestinal mucosa. Treatment involves patient education, eliminating triggers, dietary modification, and occasionally pharmacologic therapy. Consider referral to gastroenterology when red flag symptoms such as bloody stools, weight loss, family history of IBDs or colon cancer, age of presentation after 50 years, abnormal laboratory findings, or other concerning symptoms are present. Consider referral for therapy services in conjunction with medical treatment if usual medical care has not significantly improved symptoms within 3 to 6 months. Given the high prevalence of FGIDs, it is imperative that primary care physicians feel comfortable positively recognizing associated symptoms and managing the conditions, reserving referrals for extreme or prolonged cases.

CLINICS CARE POINTS

- FGIDs including IBS have negative influences on both the health and lifestyle of affected patients.
- The 2 main FGIDs are IBS and functional dyspepsia.
- Although the cause is largely unknown, immune activation after antigen presentation to intestinal mucosa may be a driving cause of clinical symptoms.
- Altered gut motility, intestinal mucosal permeability, and alterations in the microbiome may be other causes of functional gastrointestinal symptoms.
- Clinical presentation depends on the anatomic location of the patient's FGID.
- All treatment should first begin with patient education, reassurance, and setting expectations.
- Additional treatment includes eliminating triggers, dietary modification, and pharmacologic therapy in selected cases.
- Refer to gastroenterologists when red flag symptoms present or for worsening symptoms despite usual medical therapy.
- Consider referral to mental health providers if symptoms have been ongoing for at least 3 months without significant improvement from usual medical treatment alone.

DISCLOSURE

The authors have nothing to disclose.

REFERENCES

1. Sperber AD, Bangdiwala SI, Drossman DA, et al. Worldwide Prevalence and Burden of Functional Gastrointestinal Disorders, Results of Rome Foundation Global Study. Gastroenterology 2021;160:99–114.e113.
2. Ladabaum U, Boyd E, Zhao WK, et al. Diagnosis, comorbidities, and management of irritable bowel syndrome in patients in a large health maintenance organization. Clin Gastroenterol Hepatol 2012;10:37–45.
3. Lacy BE, Patel H, Guérin A, et al. Variation in Care for Patients with Irritable Bowel Syndrome in the United States. PLoS One 2016;11:e0154258.
4. Aziz I, Palsson OS, Törnblom H, et al. The Prevalence and Impact of Overlapping Rome IV-Diagnosed Functional Gastrointestinal Disorders on Somatization, Quality of Life, and Healthcare Utilization: A Cross-Sectional General Population Study in Three Countries. Am J Gastroenterol 2018;113:86–96.
5. Buono JL, Carson RT, Flores NM. Health-related quality of life, work productivity, and indirect costs among patients with irritable bowel syndrome with diarrhea. Health Qual Life Outcomes 2017;15:35.
6. Shivaji UN, Ford AC. Prevalence of functional gastrointestinal disorders among consecutive new patient referrals to a gastroenterology clinic. Frontline Gastroenterol 2014;5:266–71.
7. Bradley S, Alderson S, Ford AC, et al. General practitioners' perceptions of irritable bowel syndrome: a Q-methodological study. Fam Pract 2018;35:74–9.

8. Rocque R, Leanza Y. A Systematic Review of Patients' Experiences in Communicating with Primary Care Physicians: Intercultural Encounters and a Balance between Vulnerability and Integrity. PLoS One 2015;10:e0139577.
9. Ruddy J. From Pretending to Truly Being OK: A Journey From Illness to Health With Postinfection Irritable Bowel Syndrome: The Patient's Perspective. Gastroenterology 2018;155:1666–9.
10. Ali A, Toner BB, Stuckless N, et al. Emotional abuse, self-blame, and self-silencing in women with irritable bowel syndrome. Psychosom Med 2000;62: 76–82.
11. Drossman DA, Chang L, Schneck S, et al. A focus group assessment of patient perspectives on irritable bowel syndrome and illness severity. Dig Dis Sci 2009; 54:1532–41.
12. Palsson OS, Whitehead W, Törnblom H, et al. Prevalence of Rome IV Functional Bowel Disorders Among Adults in the United States, Canada, and the United Kingdom. Gastroenterology 2020;158:1262–73.e1263.
13. Talley NJ. What Causes Functional Gastrointestinal Disorders? A Proposed Disease Model. Am J Gastroenterol 2020;115:41–8.
14. Black CJ, Paine PA, Agrawal A, et al. British Society of Gastroenterology guidelines on the management of functional dyspepsia. Gut 2022;71:1697–723.
15. Enck P, Aziz Q, Barbara G, et al. Irritable bowel syndrome. Nat Rev Dis Primers 2016;2:16014.
16. Bischoff SC, Barbara G, Buurman W, et al. Intestinal permeability–a new target for disease prevention and therapy. BMC Gastroenterol 2014;14:189.
17. Bertiaux-Vandaële N, Youmba SB, Belmonte L, et al. The expression and the cellular distribution of the tight junction proteins are altered in irritable bowel syndrome patients with differences according to the disease subtype. Am J Gastroenterol 2011;106:2165–73.
18. Coëffier M, Gloro R, Boukhettala N, et al. Increased proteasome-mediated degradation of occludin in irritable bowel syndrome. Am J Gastroenterol 2010;105: 1181–8.
19. Martínez C, Lobo B, Pigrau M, et al. Diarrhoea-predominant irritable bowel syndrome: an organic disorder with structural abnormalities in the jejunal epithelial barrier. Gut 2013;62:1160–8.
20. Piche T, Barbara G, Aubert P, et al. Impaired intestinal barrier integrity in the colon of patients with irritable bowel syndrome: involvement of soluble mediators. Gut 2009;58:196–201.
21. Vanheel H, Vicario M, Vanuytsel T, et al. Impaired duodenal mucosal integrity and low-grade inflammation in functional dyspepsia. Gut 2014;63:262–71.
22. Valentin N, Camilleri M, Altayar O, et al. Biomarkers for bile acid diarrhoea in functional bowel disorder with diarrhoea: a systematic review and meta-analysis. Gut 2016;65:1951–9.
23. Barbara G, Cremon C, Carini G, et al. The immune system in irritable bowel syndrome. J Neurogastroenterol Motil 2011;17:349–59.
24. Barbara G, Cremon C, Annese V, et al. Randomised controlled trial of mesalazine in IBS. Gut 2016;65:82–90.
25. Lam C, Tan W, Leighton M, et al. A mechanistic multicentre, parallel group, randomised placebo-controlled trial of mesalazine for the treatment of IBS with diarrhoea (IBS-D). Gut 2016;65:91–9.
26. Barbara G, Stanghellini V, De Giorgio R, et al. Activated mast cells in proximity to colonic nerves correlate with abdominal pain in irritable bowel syndrome. Gastroenterology 2004;126:693–702.

27. Barbara G, Wang B, Stanghellini V, et al. Mast cell-dependent excitation of visceral-nociceptive sensory neurons in irritable bowel syndrome. Gastroenterology 2007;132:26–37.

28. Buhner S, Li Q, Vignali S, et al. Activation of human enteric neurons by supernatants of colonic biopsy specimens from patients with irritable bowel syndrome. Gastroenterology 2009;137:1425–34.

29. Annaházi A, Gecse K, Dabek M, et al. Fecal proteases from diarrheic-IBS and ulcerative colitis patients exert opposite effect on visceral sensitivity in mice. Pain 2009;144:209–17.

30. Annaházi A, Ferrier L, Bézirard V, et al. Luminal cysteine-proteases degrade colonic tight junction structure and are responsible for abdominal pain in constipation-predominant IBS. Am J Gastroenterol 2013;108:1322–31.

31. Valdez-Morales EE, Overington J, Guerrero-Alba R, et al. Sensitization of peripheral sensory nerves by mediators from colonic biopsies of diarrhea-predominant irritable bowel syndrome patients: a role for PAR2. Am J Gastroenterol 2013;108: 1634–43.

32. Cenac N, Bautzova T, Le Faouder P, et al. Quantification and Potential Functions of Endogenous Agonists of Transient Receptor Potential Channels in Patients With Irritable Bowel Syndrome. Gastroenterology 2015;149:433–44.e437.

33. Hughes PA, Harrington AM, Castro J, et al. Sensory neuro-immune interactions differ between irritable bowel syndrome subtypes. Gut 2013;62:1456–65.

34. Dothel G, Barbaro MR, Boudin H, et al. Nerve fiber outgrowth is increased in the intestinal mucosa of patients with irritable bowel syndrome. Gastroenterology 2015;148:1002–11.e1004.

35. Parthasarathy G, Chen J, Chen X, et al. Relationship Between Microbiota of the Colonic Mucosa vs Feces and Symptoms, Colonic Transit, and Methane Production in Female Patients With Chronic Constipation. Gastroenterology 2016;150: 367–79.e361.

36. Kassinen A, Krogius-Kurikka L, Mäkivuokko H, et al. The fecal microbiota of irritable bowel syndrome patients differs significantly from that of healthy subjects. Gastroenterology 2007;133:24–33.

37. De Palma G, Lynch M, Lu J, et al. Tu1797 The Adoptive Transfer of Anxiety and Gut Dysfunction From IBS Patients to Axenic Mice Through Microbiota Transplantation. Gastroenterology 2014;146. S-845.

38. Crouzet L, Gaultier E, Del'Homme C, et al. The hypersensitivity to colonic distension of IBS patients can be transferred to rats through their fecal microbiota. Neuro Gastroenterol Motil 2013;25:e272–82.

39. Ghaffari P, Shoaie S, Nielsen LK. Irritable bowel syndrome and microbiome; Switching from conventional diagnosis and therapies to personalized interventions. J Transl Med 2022;20:173.

40. Arpaia N, Campbell C, Fan X, et al. Metabolites produced by commensal bacteria promote peripheral regulatory T-cell generation. Nature 2013;504:451–5.

41. Shepherd SJ, Parker FC, Muir JG, et al. Dietary triggers of abdominal symptoms in patients with irritable bowel syndrome: randomized placebo-controlled evidence. Clin Gastroenterol Hepatol 2008;6:765–71.

42. Rajilić-Stojanović M, Biagi E, Heilig HG, et al. Global and deep molecular analysis of microbiota signatures in fecal samples from patients with irritable bowel syndrome. Gastroenterology 2011;141:1792–801.

43. Mayer EA, Bushnell MC. Pain IaftSo Functional pain syndromes: presentation and pathophysiology. Washington, DC: IASP Press; 2009.

44. Kano M, Dupont P, Aziz Q, et al. Understanding Neurogastroenterology From Neuroimaging Perspective: A Comprehensive Review of Functional and Structural Brain Imaging in Functional Gastrointestinal Disorders. J Neurogastroenterol Motil 2018;24:512–27.

45. Lee IS, Wang H, Chae Y, et al. Functional neuroimaging studies in functional dyspepsia patients: a systematic review. Neuro Gastroenterol Motil 2016;28:793–805.

46. Black CJ, Drossman DA, Talley NJ, et al. Functional gastrointestinal disorders: advances in understanding and management. Lancet 2020;396:1664–74.

47. Bisschops R, Karamanolis G, Arts J, et al. Relationship between symptoms and ingestion of a meal in functional dyspepsia. Gut 2008;57:1495–503.

48. Altomare A, Di Rosa C, Imperia E, et al. Diarrhea Predominant-Irritable Bowel Syndrome (IBS-D): Effects of Different Nutritional Patterns on Intestinal Dysbiosis and Symptoms. Nutrients 2021;13.

49. Drossman DA. The functional gastrointestinal disorders and the Rome II process. Gut 1999;45(Suppl 2):Ii1–5.

50. Marsh A, Eslick EM, Eslick GD. Does a diet low in FODMAPs reduce symptoms associated with functional gastrointestinal disorders? A comprehensive systematic review and meta-analysis. Eur J Nutr 2016;55:897–906.

51. Drossman DA, Ruddy J. Improving Patient-Provider Relationships to Improve Health Care. Clin Gastroenterol Hepatol 2020;18:1417–26.

52. Thompson WG, Longstreth GF, Drossman DA, et al. Functional bowel disorders and functional abdominal pain. Gut 1999;45(Suppl 2):Ii43–7.

53. Longstreth GF, Thompson WG, Chey WD, et al. Functional bowel disorders. Gastroenterology 2006;130:1480–91.

54. Fikree A, Byrne P. Management of functional gastrointestinal disorders. Clin Med 2021;21:44–52.

55. Drossman DA. Functional gastrointestinal disorders: history, pathophysiology, clinical features and Rome IV. Gastroenterology 2016;150(6):1262–79.e2.

56. Philpott HL, Nandurkar S, Lubel J, et al. Drug-induced gastrointestinal disorders. Frontline Gastroenterol 2014;5:49–57.

57. Drossman DA, Chang L. Rome IV diagnostic algorithms for common GI symptoms. Raleigh, NC: Rome Foundation; 2016.

58. Hidalgo DF, Phemister J, Ordoñez ACO, et al. Carnett's Sign: An Easy Tool That Saves Unnecessary Expenses in the Evaluation of Chronic Abdominal Pain: 1402. Official journal of the American College of Gastroenterology | ACG 2017;112:S760–1.

59. Walsham NE, Sherwood RA. Fecal calprotectin in inflammatory bowel disease. Clin Exp Gastroenterol 2016;9:21–9.

60. Labanski A, Langhorst J, Engler H, et al. Stress and the brain-gut axis in functional and chronic-inflammatory gastrointestinal diseases: A transdisciplinary challenge. Psychoneuroendocrinology 2020;111:104501.

61. Lacy BE, Pimentel M, Brenner DM, et al. ACG Clinical Guideline: Management of Irritable Bowel Syndrome. Am J Gastroenterol 2021;116:17–44.

62. Ford AC, Lacy BE, Harris LA, et al. Effect of Antidepressants and Psychological Therapies in Irritable Bowel Syndrome: An Updated Systematic Review and Meta-Analysis. Am J Gastroenterol 2019;114:21–39.

63. Keefer L, Palsson OS, Pandolfino JE. Best Practice Update: Incorporating Psychogastroenterology Into Management of Digestive Disorders. Gastroenterology 2018;154:1249–57.

64. Altobelli E, Del Negro V, Angeletti PM, et al. Low-FODMAP Diet Improves Irritable Bowel Syndrome Symptoms: A Meta-Analysis. Nutrients 2017;9.
65. Böhn L, Störsrud S, Liljebo T, et al. Diet low in FODMAPs reduces symptoms of irritable bowel syndrome as well as traditional dietary advice: a randomized controlled trial. Gastroenterology 2015;149:1399–407.e1392.
66. Barbaro MR, Cremon C, Wrona D, et al. Non-Celiac Gluten Sensitivity in the Context of Functional Gastrointestinal Disorders. Nutrients 2020;12.
67. Johannesson E, Simrén M, Strid H, et al. Physical activity improves symptoms in irritable bowel syndrome: a randomized controlled trial. Am J Gastroenterol 2011; 106:915–22.
68. Chapman RW, Stanghellini V, Geraint M, et al. Randomized clinical trial: macrogol/PEG 3350 plus electrolytes for treatment of patients with constipation associated with irritable bowel syndrome. Am J Gastroenterol 2013;108:1508–15.
69. Drossman DA, Chey WD, Johanson JF, et al. Clinical trial: lubiprostone in patients with constipation-associated irritable bowel syndrome–results of two randomized, placebo-controlled studies. Aliment Pharmacol Ther 2009;29:329–41.
70. Rao S, Lembo AJ, Shiff SJ, et al. A 12-week, randomized, controlled trial with a 4-week randomized withdrawal period to evaluate the efficacy and safety of linaclotide in irritable bowel syndrome with constipation. Am J Gastroenterol 2012;107: 1714–24 [quiz: p.1725].
71. Lembo A, Sultan S, Chang L, et al. AGA Clinical Practice Guideline on the Pharmacological Management of Irritable Bowel Syndrome With Diarrhea. Gastroenterology 2022;163:137–51.
72. Moayyedi P, Lacy BE, Andrews CN, et al. ACG and CAG Clinical Guideline: Management of Dyspepsia. Am J Gastroenterol 2017;112:988–1013.
73. Ford AC, Mahadeva S, Carbone MF, et al. Functional dyspepsia. Lancet 2020; 396:1689–702.
74. Drossman DA, Thompson WG. The irritable bowel syndrome: review and a graduated multicomponent treatment approach. Ann Intern Med 1992;116:1009–16.
75. Moayyedi P, Ford AC, Talley NJ, et al. The efficacy of probiotics in the treatment of irritable bowel syndrome: a systematic review. Gut 2010;59:325–32.
76. Brandt LJ, Chey WD, Foxx-Orenstein AE, et al. An evidence-based position statement on the management of irritable bowel syndrome. Am J Gastroenterol 2009; 104(Suppl 1):S1–35.
77. Palsson OS, Whitehead WE. Psychological treatments in functional gastrointestinal disorders: a primer for the gastroenterologist. Clin Gastroenterol Hepatol 2013;11:208–16 [quiz: e222-203].

Approach to Diarrhea

Allison Ferris, MD[a],*, Polina Gaisinskaya, MD[b],
Neilanjan Nandi, MD[c]

KEYWORDS

- Diarrhea • Primary care • Acute diarrhea • Chronic diarrhea

KEY POINTS

- History is a critical component in the evaluation of a complaint of diarrhea.
- Acute diarrhea is often self-limited and does not require specific workup or treatment, but clinicians must maintain clinical suspicion for potential life-threatening causes in the right circumstances.
- Chronic diarrhea can be more challenging but requires careful history and specific workup to reveal underlying cause.
- Utilization of gastrointestinal consultants is indicated when basic workup is unrevealing.

INTRODUCTION

Diarrhea is a common complaint in primary care offices often affecting the patient's quality of life and increasing health care resource utilization. Although most cases of diarrhea are acute and self-limiting, there are multiple causes that can lead to serious morbidity and mortality. Likewise, chronic diarrhea can be a sign of a more serious condition and requires thoughtful evaluation. Ultimately, primary care physicians must take an evidence-based and comprehensive approach to diarrhea to appropriately apply health care resources in the interest of patient care.

PREVALENCE AND INCIDENCE

Worldwide, acute diarrhea affects more than one billion people per year, with 90% of cases being infectious in origin.[1] In the United States, nearly 179 million people experience acute diarrhea at least once per year, with nearly 10% of them consulting a health care provider and 500,000 ending up hospitalized for their diarrheal illness.[2,3]

[a] Internal Medicine Residency Program, Department of Medicine, Charles E. Schmidt College of Medicine, Florida Atlantic University, 800 Meadows Road, Boca Raton, FL 33486, USA; [b] Internal Medicine Residency Program, Department of Medicine, Charles E. Schmidt College of Medicine, Graduate Medical Education Consortium, Bethesda Hospital, Boca Raton Regional Hospital, Delray Medical Center, Florida Atlantic University, 800 Meadows Road, Boca Raton, FL 33486, USA, [c] Division of Gastroenterology and Hepatology, Perelman School of Medicine, University of Pennsylvania, 3737 Market Street, 11th floor, Philadelphia, PA 19104, USA
* Corresponding author.
E-mail address: ferrisa@health.fau.edu

Prim Care Clin Office Pract 50 (2023) 447–459
https://doi.org/10.1016/j.pop.2023.03.010
0095-4543/23/© 2023 Elsevier Inc. All rights reserved.
primarycare.theclinics.com

More than 5000 people die each year in the United States from acute diarrheal illness and its complications.[2,3] One group of researchers surveyed people by phone to better determine the prevalence of diarrhea in the United States. This study revealed an overall prevalence of 7.7% (incidence of 0.6 episodes/person/year), with 19.5% visiting a medical provider at least once.[4]

Incidence and prevalence of chronic diarrhea is a bit more challenging to measure, as people often adapt to their condition and may not seek medical care.[5] A study based on NHANES data in 2009 to 2010 attempted to better measure the prevalence of chronic diarrhea in the United States using Bristol stool chart 6 or 7 and estimates 6.6% prevalence of chronic diarrhea.[6] In general, most estimates indicate chronic diarrhea has a prevalence of 2% to 7%,[1,5] which is observed to increase to as much as 7% to 14% when focusing on an elderly patient demographic.[5]

The health care economic cost of diarrhea including lost wages and productivity has been estimated to be ∼ 8 billion dollars per year.[1]

PATHOPHYSIOLOGY

Diarrhea can be defined in various ways. The purest definition is an increase in stool water content or frequency such that stool weight is greater than 200 g per day.[1] Because this measurement is not practiced, an easier definition is the one used by the World Health Organization that defines diarrhea as 3 or more liquid stools in a 24-hour period.[3] The Bristol Stool Chart is a visual representation of stool appearance that corresponds to gut transit time, with stool types 5 to 7 being representative of shortened gut transit time and therefore characterized as diarrhea.[5,7]

The temporal duration of diarrhea, categorized as acute versus chronic in nature, can affect the approach to management. Acute diarrhea lasts less than 2 weeks and chronic diarrhea lasts greater than 4 weeks.[1,8] Diarrhea lasting between 2 and 4 weeks is considered persistent diarrhea.[1,8]

Ninety percent of acute diarrhea is infectious in origin,[1] with norovirus as the predominant cause in 58% of cases.[3,9] Acute diarrhea has several causes such as fecal-oral, food/water borne, and disturbance of the normal gastrointestinal (GI) flora.[1] Travelers diarrhea affects up to 40% of visitors to destinations in Latin America, Africa, and Asia,[1] resulting in between 4 and 17 million cases each year.[8] Food-borne organisms represent a major source of acute infectious diarrhea, with approximately 48 million people affected per year.[8] Most of the food-borne acute diarrhea is related to produce, with leafy green vegetables as the predominant culprit.[9]

Acute infectious diarrhea is often self-limiting[3] and is associated with the following:

- Fever
- Nausea
- Abdominal pain
- Bloating
- Gas
- Tenesmus
- Fecal urgency[1,8]

Acute watery diarrhea is often secondary to small bowel hypersecretion as a result of preformed toxins created by bacteria or by bacteria that adhere to the bowel mucosa.[1] Bloody diarrhea in the acute setting is not common (only 3.5% of respondents reported blood),[4] but it often represents an inflammatory infectious cause[2,3] due to a host of causes that commonly include *Salmonella, Campylobacter, Clostridium difficile, Shigella, and Shiga toxin–producing Escherichia coli*.[2,3] Risk of death from acute infectious diarrhea is highest with Salmonella.[2,3,9] Common food-borne bacterial infections are shown in **Fig. 1**.

The remaining 10% of acute diarrhea is caused by medications, toxins, ischemia, or food (such as lactose intolerance) as shown in **Fig. 2**.[1]

Common medication culprits include the following:

- Antibiotics (especially macrolides)
- Antiarrhythmics (such as quinidine, β-blockers)
- Antihypertensives (angiotensin-converting enzyme inhibitors)
- Nonsteroidal anti-inflammatory drugs (cyclooxygenase 1 inhibitors)
- Antidepressants (sertraline)
- Chemotherapy agents
- Antacids (proton pump inhibitors)
- Bronchodilators (beta-2 agonists)
- Laxatives[1]

In addition to the diarrhea patients experience as a result of chemotherapy, patients with graft-versus-host disease can present with acute diarrhea. Acute ischemic colitis can present with an episode of abdominal pain followed by diarrhea, usually watery first, then bloody later.[1]

Chronic diarrhea has a wide variety of causes including the following:

- Malignancy
- Inflammation
- Pancreatic insufficiency
- Motility disorders[5]

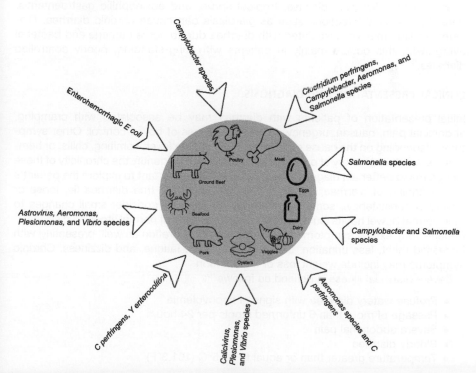

Fig. 1. Common food-borne bacterial infections.

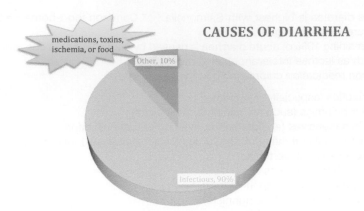

CAUSES OF DIARRHEA

medications, toxins, ischemia, or food

Other, 10%

Infectious, 90%

Fig. 2. Causes of acute diarrhea.

Less common causes of chronic diarrhea include small intestinal bacterial overgrowth (SIBO), chronic mesenteric ischemia, postsurgical changes, radiation enteropathy, hyperthyroidism, cystic fibrosis, diabetes mellitus, and chronic pancreatitis.[5] It is important to note that some conditions can initially seem as acute diarrhea but after time will reveal themselves as a chronic cause, such as is often seen with the initial presentation of inflammatory bowel disease. Malabsorption can be due to enzymatic deficiency of specific sugars (lactose, fructose, sucrose) or malabsorption of nonabsorbable sugars (xylitol, maltitol, mannitol, sorbitol). Other rare causes include Whipple disease, tropical sprue, and eosinophilic gastroenteritis. Parasitic intestinal infections such as giardiasis can cause chronic diarrhea. Diabetes mellitus may be associated with diarrhea due to nerve damage and bacterial overgrowth; this occurs mainly in patients with long-standing, poorly controlled diabetes.[9]

CLINICAL PRESENTATION AND DIAGNOSIS

Initial presentation of patients with diarrhea may be associated with cramping, abdominal pain, nausea, urgency, tenesmus, or loss of bowel control. Other symptoms, depending on the cause of diarrhea, may include fever, vomiting, chills, or hematochezia.[10] Initial history at presentation is important to identify the chronicity of these symptoms to better aid diagnostic workup. It is also important to explore the patient's understanding of diarrhea; although they may describe true diarrhea (ie, loose or watery in consistency), some patients may erroneously consider small changes to their normal bowel habits (such as increased frequency of normal stool) as diarrhea.[11] Patients may exhibit symptoms associated with dehydration as well, presenting with increased thirst, less urination, dark urine, dry skin, fatigue, and dizziness. Chronic symptoms may include weight loss or malnutrition.

Severe diarrheal illness is defined as follows[10]:

- Profuse watery diarrhea with signs of hypovolemia
- Passage of more than 6 unformed stools per 24 hours
- Severe abdominal pain
- Bloody diarrhea
- Temperature greater than or equal to 38.5°C (101.3°F)

Alarm features include the following[12]:

- Onset after age 50 years
- Hematochezia or melena
- Nocturnal pain/diarrhea
- Unexplained weight loss
- Laboratory abnormalities (iron deficiency anemia, elevated C-reactive protein, or fecal calprotectin)
- Family history of inflammatory bowel disease (IBD) or colorectal cancer

It is also important to keep in mind concomitant risk factors for deterioration of patients, particularly the elderly, immunocompromised, pregnant women, and those with significant exposure risk.[13]

Initial studies based on history may include the following:

- Complete blood count
- Complete metabolic panel, including albumin for nutritional status
- Thyroid hormone panel
- Vitamin and mineral testing (iron, B12, folate, 25-hydroxyvitamin D)
- Inflammatory markers such as erythrocyte sedimentation rate, C-reactive protein, and fecal calprotectin
- Stool culture, ova and parasite test, C difficile screening.
- Shiga toxin (due to risk of development of hemolytic uremic syndrome)
- Stool rotavirus antigen testing by enzyme immunoassay and latex agglutination

FURTHER TESTING

Stool studies for fecal fat, microscopic amounts of blood, and white blood cells will help determine if diarrhea is fatty or inflammatory. Specifically, fecal calprotectin is more sensitive for colonic inflammation than small bowel disease and can sometimes help differentiate between IBD and irritable bowel syndrome (IBS); this can further aid in pinpointing the location of mucosal disruption, small versus large bowel as mentioned in **Table 1**. Hydrogen breath testing may aid in diagnosing lactose intolerance.[12,13]

Table 1
Common infections, their presenting characteristics, and diagnostic results

	Small Bowel	Large Bowel
Consistency	Watery	Mucoid/grossly bloody
Volume	Large	Small
Frequency	Increased	Excessively increased
Leukocytosis	None	Present
Pathogens	• Rotavirus • Adenovirus • Calicivirus • Astrovirus • Norovirus • E coli • Klebsiella • Clostridium perfringens • Cholera species • Vibrio species • Giardia species • Cryptosporidium species	• Escherichia coli (enteroinvasive, enterohemorrhagic) • Shigella species • Salmonella species • Campylobacter species • Yersinia species • Aeromonas species • Plesiomonas species • Clostridium difficile • Entamoeba organisms

If there is suspicion for celiac disease/sprue, IBD, IBS, small bowel bacterial overgrowth, pancreatic insufficiency, or malignancy, then additional evaluation including referral to a GI physician may be indicated.

Imaging should be reserved for patients with peritoneal signs, usually warranting an abdominopelvic computed tomography (CT), when possible. When appropriate, the presence of constitutional signs or symptoms or refractory abdominal pain may also warrant cross-sectional imaging consideration. In addition, emergent evaluation and surgical consultation should be considered.

TREATMENT
General Guidelines

Regardless of the duration of diarrhea, the initial approach should be directed at evaluation and management of hydration status and dietary counseling. Severe, acute infectious diarrhea can often lead to greater physiologic stress by depleting whole-body volume rapidly. Home-based oral hydration is appropriate when dehydration is of mild to moderate severity. Appropriate use of rehydration solutions is critical to not worsening the patient's clinical status. Enteral rehydration requires cotransport of glucose and sodium, which necessitates rehydration solutions composed of equimolar concentrations of these components. When these are not balanced, then dehydration can be exacerbated. For instance, some common commercial sports drink rehydration solutions contain a high carbohydrate load to low sodium content ratio, which may increase osmotic diarrhea. Another commonly used solution, high sodium chicken or beef broth, may promote diarrheal volume losses that contribute to the development of hypernatremia. Fortunately, rehydration solutions can be homemade or available at pharmacies (eg, Pedialyte). Orthostatic symptoms and vitals, poor skin turgor, and dry mucous membranes can herald severe dehydration, which may best benefit from intravenous hydration with normal saline or lactated Ringer solution.

Active nausea or vomiting may require temporary *nil per os* (NPO) status, which may be therapeutic in allowing an infectious organism to run its course and permit the body's purge of diarrheal toxin. During acute diarrhea, some foods may be challenging to digest and process. For instance, active enteritis can cause a temporary loss of lactase along the brush border, which can promote some relative increase in temporary dairy intolerance. Therefore, temporary cessation of lactose-containing products may help reduce diarrheal volume loss. Also, low-starch, low-sodium diets (eg, BRAT diet) consisting of bananas, rice, applesauce, and toast may temporarily help patients manage their symptoms acutely. **Table 2** summarizes several common treatment regimens

Infectious Causes

Most causes of infectious diarrhea, including Travelers diarrhea and many bacterial culprits, will resolve within a few days without antibiotic requirement. When this diarrhea is unremitting, empiric treatment with antibiotics may be necessary. Antibiotic options may include rifaximin, which belongs to the rifamycin class that has poor intestinal absorption and, therefore, limits systemic toxicity. This contrasts with quinolones that carry greater adverse event profile and promote antibiotic resistance. Azithromycin is another effective option in treating Travelers diarrhea as well.

Indeed, indiscriminate antibiotic administration can destroy beneficial bacteria, leading to intestinal dysbiosis and antibiotic-associated diarrhea, a portion of which can include *C difficile*. Antibiotics can also promote selection for resistant strains of

Table 2
Treatment regimens

Cause	Treatment Recommendation	Dose/Duration
Travelers diarrhea	Azithromycin	1000 mg po once OR 500 mg po daily x 3d
	Rifaximin	200 mg po tid x 3d
	Rifamycin	2 (194 mg) tablets po bid x 3d
	Levofloxacin	500 mg po daily (1d OR 3d)
	Ciprofloxacin	750 mg po once OR 500 mg po bid x 3d
	Ofloxacin	400 mg po daily (1d OR 3d)
Confirmed or suspected STEC (E coli O157:H7 or non-O157:H7)	Consider discontinuing antibiotics due to concern of HUS	N/A
C difficile	Nonsevere disease	
	• Vancomycin	125 mg po qid x 10d
	• Fidaxomicin	200 mg po bid x 10d
	• Alternate treatment if aforementioned not available	
	• Metronidazole	500 mg po tid x 10–14d
	Severe C difficile	
	• PO + PR vancomycin and consider adjunctive metronidazole IV	
Prevention of recurrent C difficile	Bezlotoxumab antitoxin IV infusion	Single dose at 10 mg/kg over 50 min
	RBX2660 (REBYOTA)	Administer rectal enema w/in 24–72 h postantibiotic completion
	Fecal microbiota transplantation (FMT)	Non–FDA-approved consult GI/ID w/FMT expertise
Bile acid diarrhea	Cholestyramine	2 g po daily or bid (can titrate up as needed)
	Colestipol	2–16 g/d po divided up to qid (if tablets) 5–30 g/d po divided up to qid (if granules)
	Colesevelam	1.875 g po bid
SIBO	Rifaximin	550 mg po tid x 14d
	Methanogen predominant	Neomycin, 500 mg, po bid x 14d
	• Rifaximin + neomycin	

Abbreviation: HUS, hemolytic uremic syndrome.

extended-spectrum beta-lactamase *E coli* and other multidrug-resistant organisms. Treatment of *enterohemorrhagic E coli* with antibiotics can potentiate the development of hemolytic uremic syndrome. Therefore, the appropriate application of antibiotics is typically necessary when clinical sequelae include fever, copious purulent mucus, or severe abdominal pain. Antidiarrheals may be deployed judiciously to control diarrheal volume loss but should be temporarily held if abdominal pain or fever continues to worsen suggesting that bacterial endotoxin is not being purged effectively.

The treatment of *C difficile* can be challenging, especially in an antibiotic prescription era that can potentiate further recurrence. Importantly, metronidazole is not a preferred first-line agent in *C difficile* treatment. Fidaxomicin and vancomycin both have similar rates of efficacy but meta-analyses and head-to-head studies have shown that fidaxomicin treatment is associated with less risk of recurrence than vancomycin.[14,15] For patients with nonsevere *C difficile* infection an initial 10-day course of fidaxomicin or vancomycin is effective.[16] Patients with a first recurrence of *C difficile* can be retreated with fidaxomicin or a course of vancomycin (standard, pulsed dose, or extended taper). Indeed, vancomycin tapers can help prolong some antibiotic-induced remission of germinating *C difficile* spores and help patients achieve clinical quiescence. Patients with recurrent *C difficile infection* are candidates to receive a one-time intravenous infusion of bezlotoxumab, an antitoxin that is given concomitant to antibiotics during active *C difficile* infection and has demonstrated a decrease in *C difficile* recurrence thereafter. The Food and Drug Administration (FDA) considers fecal microbiota transplantation (FMT) an investigational option that has demonstrated upward of 90% to 100% efficacy when delivered via colonoscopy.[17,18] The Infectious Diseases Society of America notes that FMT should be considered in patients with multiple *C difficile* infection recurrence who have failed other standard-of-care antibiotic therapies.[16] Case reports of pathogenic *E coli* transmission and SARS-COV-2 transmission have prompted the FDA to issue several safety alerts in recent years. To improve safety, there are several microbiome-derived therapies for *C difficile* in clinical trial development. RBX2660, a stool microbiota–derived biotherapeutic enema, was approved in November 2022 for use as a preventative measure in patients with established current *C difficile* infection.[19] It must be administered within 24 to 72 hours following *C difficile* infection for benefit.

Bile Acid Irritation

Excess bile acid irritation of the colonic mucosa can occur in conditions such as bile acid diarrhea and in the postoperative state following cholecystectomy. Treatment may require use of bile acid sequestrants (eg, cholestyramine, colestipol, colesevelam) to bind excess bile acids and improve stool consistency.

Small Intestinal Bacterial Overgrowth

Once the diagnosis of SIBO has been established, the mainstay of therapy uses antibiotics. In general, these patients benefit from rifaximin, 550 mg, po tid for 14 days. In those who have intestinal methanogen-predominant overgrowth, the combination of this rifaximin regimen with neomycin, 500 mg, twice daily for 14 days can markedly improve diarrhea.[20] Other antibiotics used to treat these conditions include quinolones, penicillins, metronidazole, tetracycline, and trimethoprim-sulfamethoxazole. However, observational studies suggest that rifaximin is very effective with less systemic side effects, in contrast to other antibiotics, due to its limited intestinal absorption into the systemic circulation.[21]

Irritable Bowel Syndrome with Diarrhea

Notably, there is a broad paucity of studies regarding IBS mixed phenotype although there are several treatment modalities focused on treating IBS with diarrhea predominance. In recent years, an abundance of data has supported the efficacy of gut-directed hypnotherapy and cognitive behavioral therapy for patients with IBS.[22–24] Patients with particular dietary sensitivities and abdominal distention may benefit from a diet low in fermentable oligosaccharide, disaccharide, monosaccharide, and polyols (low FODMAPs). Specific components of the FODMOP diet are discussed more in depth in Molly Duffy and colleagues' article, "Functional Gastrointestinal Disorders," in this issue.

Fiber plays a complex role in gut microbiota metabolism and human health. Specifically, soluble fibers that are more viscous and less fermentable (such as oat, bran, barley, beans and psyllium husk), have demonstrated increased stool consistency in patients with IBS-D.[25] A long-used therapy has been peppermint oil (*Mentha piperita*), which has demonstrable effects on smooth muscle relaxation throughout the entire intestinal tract. Although nonencapsulated peppermint oil may relax lower esophageal sphincter tone leading to gastroesophageal reflux disease, encapsulated small bowel release preparations have demonstrated decreased abdominal discomfort in comparison to placebo, thus serving as a low-risk option with evidence-based therapeutic effect.[26]

Indeed, the role of gut microbiota in GI illness is a significant area of therapeutic interest. It has been observed that following an acute gastroenteritis, approximately 20% to 30% of patients may develop a dysbiosis that is clinically recognized as post-infectious IBS-D. This can be effectively treated with rifaximin and has become a mainstay of treatment as a result of trials of rifaximin, 550 mg, t.i.d. for 2 weeks, demonstrating that one round of treatment can improve abdominal pain and improve stool consistency, with a second round of treatment improving both urgency and bloating.[27] Probiotics supplementation in IBS-D has not demonstrated benefit, and fecal microbiota transplantation interventional studies have been observed with mixed results necessitating the need for more high-quality investigational studies.

Patients with IBS-D may also benefit from various symptomatic treatments, with those patients with IBS-D who remain incompletely treated potentially benefitting from more chronic daily therapy. This is discussed further in Molly Duffy and colleagues' article, "Functional Gastrointestinal Disorders," in this issue.

Immune-Mediated Diarrhea

Immune-mediated causes of diarrhea include celiac disease, eosinophilic gastrointestinal disease (EGID), and IBD. The mainstay of celiac treatment begins with gluten restriction and working with a dietitian to ensure that nutritional stores are repleted and optimized. Current management of EGIDs involves pursuing a 6-food elimination diet (eggs, wheat, soy, dairy, shellfish, nuts) even without esophageal involvement, although many adult patients will not necessarily respond to these interventions adequately. A trial of systemic corticosteroids (eg, prednisone) may be required. For recurrent disease, some patients may require transition to immediate or extended-release budesonide depending on the location of their disease (ileum- and proximal colon vs colon, respectively). In recent years, patients with Crohn and ulcerative colitis have benefited from an ever-expanding treatment armamentarium.

Pancreatic Insufficiency–Associated Diarrhea

Pancreatic insufficiency can be markedly improved with enteric-coated pancreatic enzyme supplementation. The amount of enzymatic capsule supplementation is titrated to the patient's dietary intake of fat and symptoms. Patients who restrict pork products from their diet should be informed that the lipase is commonly porcine derived.

Medication-Induced Diarrhea

The list of culprits mediating medication-induced diarrhea is long. Careful history taking as to the onset of diarrhea and changes in medication start, dosing, or frequency are necessary to suspecting temporal causation. Discontinuing the medication, and when necessary, rechallenge of the offending medication may be necessary to demonstrate causation.

Chronic Diarrhea

In clinical practice, the hunt for culprit chronic diarrheal causes may eventually diagnose chronic infections with protozoan parasite giardiasis; this can be effectively treated with small doses of metronidazole, nitazoxanide, or paromomycin. Helminthic infections commonly occur with whipworm or hookworm and are often underdiagnosed. Fortunately, antihelminthic therapy with albendazole, mebendazole, or ivermectin can be promptly effective. Immunocompromised patients may be susceptible to opportunistic infection with *Cyclospora* and *Cystoisospora* and be effectively treated with trimethoprim-sulfamethoxazole. *Microsporidial* infection can be treated with albendazole or fumagillin.

Indications for gastroenterology referral

When initial laboratory and stool testing are unrevealing and empiric interventions such as lactose restriction or antibiotics fail to relieve symptoms, referral to a gastroenterologist should be considered for further cognitive consultation and, if deemed necessary, endoscopic assessment (**Fig. 3**). The presence of alarm or constitutional signs or symptoms including new onset of fevers, chills, and unintentional weight

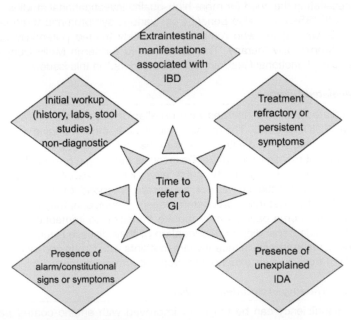

Fig. 3. Indications for gastroenterology referral.

loss should signal early triage to GI consultation. A review of systems may occasionally reveal extraintestinal manifestations (EIMs) of IBD. Four such EIMs that can parallel intestinal disease activity include the presence of oral aphthous ulcers, anterior uveitis, inflammatory arthralgia, and erythema nodosum.

GI consultants can directly visualize the bowel through upper endoscopy, colonoscopy, or enteroscopy in either anterograde or retrograde routes to assess the small bowel. Consultants can also perform specific small bowel evaluation with video capsule endoscopy for identifying occult GI bleeding cause or inflammation. Although imaging modalities can be requested by any clinician, GI consultants can expertly identify when MR/CT enterography imaging is necessary to evaluate the small bowel for pathology. Notably, noninvasive breath testing to assess for fermentative organisms can also be interpreted by GI consultants as well. Advanced interventional endoscopists also provide a skill set that can assess the hepatobiliary tree for occult tumors or pancreatic insufficiency in certain unique situations as well.

CLINICS CARE POINTS

- Gathering a history should include information about food exposures, but it is also important to gauge risk of severe disease or inflammatory conditions, suggested by bloody stool, abdominal pain, fever, weight loss, and/or hypovolemia from profuse watery diarrhea.

- Fecal calprotectin may help differentiate functional disease (eg, IBS) from inflammatory disease of the colon (eg, IBD).

- Metronidazole is no longer a first-line agent for treatment of *C difficile*. Although fidaxomicin and vancomycin are equally efficacious in the treatment of *C difficile*, fidaxomicin is associated with reduced risk of recurrence posttreatment.

- IBS with bloating or diarrheal predominance may benefit from low FODMAP approach to dietary modification.

FUNDING SOURCES

The authors have no funding to declare.

CONFLICTS OF INTEREST

Dr N. Nandi has served as a consult and advisor to Boehringer-Ingelheim, Bristol Myers Squibb, Janssen & Janssen, and Pfizer.

REFERENCES

1. Camilleri M, Murray JA. Diarrhea and constipation. In: Loscalzo J, Fauci A, Kasper D, et al, editors. Harrison's Principles of Internal Medicine, 21e. McGraw Hill; 2022. Available at: https://accessmedicine-mhmedical-com.ezproxy.fau.edu/content.aspx?bookid=3095&sectionid=262790621. Accessed August 16, 2022.
2. Meisenheimer ES, Epstein C, Thiel D. Acute diarrhea in adults. Am Fam Physician 2022 Jul;106(1):72–80. PMID: 35839362.
3. Shane AL, Mody RK, Crump JA, et al. 2017 infectious diseases society of america clinical practice guidelines for the diagnosis and management of infectious diarrhea. Clin Infect Dis 2017;65(12):e45–80.

4. Jones TF, McMillian MB, Scallan E, et al. A population-based estimate of the substantial burden of diarrhoeal disease in the United States; FoodNet, 1996-2003. Epidemiol Infect 2007;135(2):293–301.

5. Arasaradnam RP, Brown S, Forbes A, et al. Guidelines for the investigation of chronic diarrhoea in adults: British Society of Gastroenterology. Gut 2018;67(8): 1380–99, 3rd ed.

6. Singh P, Mitsuhashi S, Ballou S, et al. Demographic and dietary associations of chronic diarrhea in a representative sample of adults in the United States. Am J Gastroenterol 2018;113(4):593–600.

7. O'Donnell LJ, Virjee J, Heaton KW. Detection of pseudodiarrhoea by simple clinical assessment of intestinal transit rate. BMJ 1990;300(6722):439–40.

8. Riddle MS, DuPont HL, Connor BA. ACG clinical guideline: diagnosis, treatment, and prevention of acute diarrheal infections in adults. Am J Gastroenterol 2016; 111(5):602–22.

9. DuPont HL. Acute infectious diarrhea in immunocompetent adults. N Engl J Med 2014;370(16):1532–40.

10. DuPont HL. Practice Parameters Committee of the American College of Gastroenterology. Guidelines on acute infectious diarrhea in adults. Am J Gastroenterol 1997;92(11):1962–75.

11. Ramaswamy K, Jacobson K. Infectious diarrhea in children. Gastroenterol Clin North Am 2001;30(3):611–24.

12. Ochoa B and Suarwicz CM. Diarrheal Diseases-Acute and Chronic. Available at: https://gi.org/topics/diarrhea-acute-and-chronic/. Accessed October 30, 2022.

13. Nemeth V, Pfleghaar N. Diarrhea. Treasure Island (FL): StatPearls Publishing; 2022. StatPearls.

14. Al Momani LA, Abughanimeh O, Boonpheng B, et al. Fidaxomicin vs vancomycin for the treatment of a first episode of clostridium difficile infection: a meta-analysis and systematic review. Cureus 2018;10(6):e2778.

15. Louie TJ, Miller MA, Weiss K, et al. Fidaxomicin versus vancomycin for *Clostridium difficile* infection. N Engl J Med 2011;364:422–31.

16. Johnson S, Lavergne V, Skinner AM, et al. Clinical practice guideline by the infectious diseases society of America (IDSA) and society for healthcare epidemiology of America (SHEA): 2021 focused update guidelines on management of clostridioides difficile infection in adults. Clin Infect Dis 2021;73(5):e1029–44.

17. FDA Guidance to Industry: Enforcement Policy Regarding Investigational New Drug Requirements for Use of Fecal Microbiota for Transplantation to Treat Clostridium difficile Infection Not Responsive to Standard Therapies. Available at: https://www.fda.gov/media/86440/download/. Accessed November 1, 2022.

18. Aroniadis OC, Brandt LJ. Intestinal microbiota and the efficacy of fecal microbiota transplantation in gastrointestinal disease. Gastroenterol Hepatol 2014;10(4): 230–7. PMID: 24976806; PMCID: PMC4073534.

19. Khanna S, Assi M, Lee C, et al. Efficacy and safety of RBX2660 in PUNCH CD3, a phase III, randomized, double-blind, placebo-controlled trial with a bayesian primary analysis for the prevention of recurrent clostridioides difficile infection. Drugs 2022;82(15):1527–38. Epub 2022 Oct 26. Erratum in: Drugs. 2022 Nov 7;: PMID: 36287379; PMCID: PMC9607700.

20. Pimentel M, Saad RJ, Long MD, et al. ACG clinical guideline: small intestinal bacterial overgrowth. Am J Gastroenterol 2020;115(2):165–78.

21. Shayto RH, Abou Mrad R, Sharara AI. Use of rifaximin in gastrointestinal and liver diseases. World J Gastroenterol 2016;22(29):6638–51.

22. Lackner JM, Jaccard J, Radziwon CD, et al. Durability and decay of treatment benefit of cognitive behavioral therapy for irritable bowel syndrome: 12-month follow-up. Am J Gastroenterol 2019;114(2):330–8.

23. Miller V, Carruthers HR, Morris J, et al. Hypnotherapy for irritable bowel syndrome: an audit of one thousand adult patients. Aliment Pharmacol Ther 2015; 41(9):844–55.

24. Palsson OS. Hypnosis treatment of gastrointestinal disorders: a comprehensive review of the empirical evidence. Am J Clin Hypn 2015;58(2):134–58.

25. Moayyedi P, Quigley EM, Lacy BE, et al. The effect of fiber supplementation on irritable bowel syndrome: a systematic review and meta-analysis. Am J Gastroenterol 2014;109:1367–74.

26. Alammar N, Wang L, Saberi B, et al. The impact of peppermint oil on the irritable bowel syndrome: a meta-analysis of the pooled clinical data. BMC Compliment Altern Med 2019;19:21.

27. Lacy BE, Pimentel M, Brenner DM, et al. ACG clinical guideline: management of irritable bowel syndrome. Am J Gastroenterol 2021;116(1):17–44.

Benign Colorectal Disorders

Mirtha Y. Aguilar-Alvarado, MD, MPH[a,1], Bernadette Baker, MD[a,1],
Laura S. Chiu, MD, MPH[b], Megha K. Shah, MD, MSc[a,*]

KEYWORDS

- Diverticulosis • Diverticulitis • Hemorrhoids • Anal warts • Anogenital conditions

KEY POINTS

- Diverticular disease represents spectrum of conditions related to the presence of diverticula or sac-like protrusions of the colon wall; most are asymptomatic but can be associated with bleeding, infection, perforation, fistula, or obstruction.
- Hemorrhoids are characterized by the abnormal downward displacement of the anal cushions causing venous dilatation that most commonly presents as painless bleeding and intermittent protrusion.
- Anogenital warts are a common sexually transmitted epithelial growth caused by the human papillomavirus (HPV) 2. HPV types 6 and 11 account for most external anal and genital warts in male and female patients 2,3.
- Anal fissures are common superficial tears involving the anal canal that can cause significant pain during and after stooling.
- Pruritis ani, or perianal itching, is common condition is often undiagnosed due to a limited number that seek care for this socially embarrassing condition.

INTRODUCTION

Benign conditions of the colon and rectum are a heterogenous group of conditions that range from inflammatory to infectious to pelvic floor health conditions that affect large segments of the US population. These conditions include diverticular disease, hemorrhoids, and anorectal lesions. The initial presentation of these very common conditions often occurs in the outpatient primary care setting, and most can be managed by the primary care physician. This article provides an overview on the prevalence, diagnosis, and management of some of the most common benign colorectal disorders; these are broadly divided into diverticular disease, hemorrhoids, and anorectal conditions. As with all clinical evaluations, diagnosis begins with a thorough

---

[a] Department of Family and Preventive Medicine, Emory School of Medicine, Atlanta, GA, USA;
[b] Department of Medicine, Section of Gastroenterology, Boston University School of Medicine, Boston, MA, USA
[1] Present address: 4500 North Shallowford Road, Dunwoody, GA 30338.
* Corresponding author. 4500 North Shallowford Road, Dunwoody, GA 30338.
E-mail address: mkshah@emory.edu

Prim Care Clin Office Pract 50 (2023) 461–480
https://doi.org/10.1016/j.pop.2023.03.011
0095-4543/23/Published by Elsevier Inc.
primarycare.theclinics.com

history and physical examination. For each condition, this review includes additional specific evaluation tools and recommendations.

Diverticular disease represents a clinical spectrum of conditions related to the presence of diverticula, or sac-like protrusions of the colon wall. Diverticulosis, defined by the presence of diverticula, can be asymptomatic or symptomatic as a result of associated bleeding, infection, perforation, fistula, or obstruction due to chronic inflammation.

Hemorrhoids are characterized by the abnormal downward displacement of the anal cushions causing venous dilatation.[1] According to the location, hemorrhoids can be classified as internal (if proximal to the dentate line), external (if distal to the dentate line), or mixed (proximal and distal) (**Fig. 1**).

Common anorectal conditions include anogenital warts, anal fissures, and pruritis ani. Anogenital warts (AGWs) are a common sexually transmitted epithelial growth caused by the human papillomavirus (HPV).[2] HPV types 6 and 11 account for most external anal and genital warts in male and female patients.[2,3] Although AGWs are generally benign, they can be physically uncomfortable to patients and cosmetically displeasing. Anal fissures are common superficial tears involving the anal canal that can cause significant pain during and after stooling. It is commonly associated with a history of constipation and trauma to the anal canal. Other common benign anal conditions include pruritis ani, or perianal itching. This very common condition is often undiagnosed due to a limited number that seek care for this socially embarrassing condition.

DIVERTICULAR DISEASE
Prevalence

The incidence of diverticular disease notably increases with age, and has been on the rise in the United States and other industrialized societies.[4] Approximately 15% to 30% of individuals by the age of 50 years[5] and 60% to 70% by the age of 80 may be affected by diverticulosis.[5,6] Diverticulitis affects roughly 4% to 15% of patients

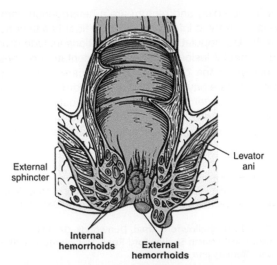

Fig. 1. The origin and location of internal and external hemorrhoids. (*From* Lewis S, et al. Medical-Surgical Nursing: Assessment and Management of Clinical Problems, ed 10. St Louis: Elsevier; 2017.)

with diverticulosis,[7] with an estimated incidence of 180/100,000 persons per year in the US population. Although older adults are most commonly affected by diverticulitis, the rate of diverticulitis among the younger adults has increased most dramatically in the recent decades.[8] Particularly, the incidence of diverticulitis in individuals 40 to 49 years has risen by 132% from 1980 to 2007.[8]

Pathophysiology

Diverticula, or abnormal sac-like outpouchings of the colon wall, are thought to occur due to the interactions of high intraluminal pressures, disordered motility, and alterations in colonic structure.[9] Diverticulosis typically develops where the vasa recta penetrate the colonic circular muscle layer, areas of relative weakness of the bowel wall. This results in the herniation of the mucosa and submucosa through the colon wall muscle layer, termed pseudodiverticulum or "false" diverticulum. Diverticulosis most commonly occurs in the sigmoid colon. This region is associated with decreased luminal diameter and hypertrophy of the muscular layers, resulting in disordered motility and increased luminal pressure that facilitates diverticulosis formation.[6]

Diverticulitis is caused by the micro- and macroscopic perforation of a colonic diverticulum (**Fig. 2**). Colon wall and peri-colonic inflammation occur as a result of feculent fluid extravasation through the ruptured diverticulum. Persistent inflammation and focal necrosis may lead to further associated complications, including abscess or perforation.[6]

Risk factors associated with increased risk of symptomatic diverticular disease include[10–13]

- High dietary intake of red meat
- Lack of vigorous physical activity
- Obesity
- Heavy smoking
- Low dietary fiber, which causes decreased bulking in colonic stool content and subsequent increased colonic pressures for feces propulsion may also increase the risk of diverticulosis[14]

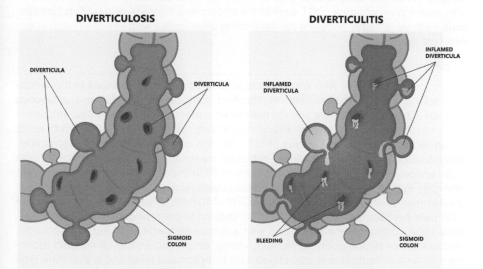

Fig. 2. Colonic diverticulosis and diverticulitis. (©Rumrauy/Adobe Stock.)

Additionally, nuts and seeds are not associated with increased risk of diverticulitis according to an updated large observational study,[15] despite historical perspective. Genetic predisposition is an associated factor as well, contributing up to 50% of the risk for diverticulitis.[16]

Clinical Presentation

Diverticulosis is asymptomatic in the majority of patients, as it is often found incidentally on imaging or endoscopy. Diverticulosis becomes symptomatic if it is associated with further issues, including infection.

Diverticulitis typically presents with the acute or subacute onset of abdominal pain. Abdominal tenderness on palpation during physical examination is most commonly located in the left lower quadrant due to the involvement of the sigmoid colon. It can be accompanied by fevers, nausea, vomiting, altered bowel habits, anorexia, and urinary complaints if there is concomitant inflammation of the bladder. The severity and symptoms of diverticulitis depend on the degree of inflammation. Most acute diverticulitis cases are uncomplicated. However, approximately 12% of patients with diverticulitis are considered complicated,[17,18] associated with the presence of phlegmon or abscess, peritonitis, obstruction, stricture, or fistula. Physical examination may demonstrate a tender mass if there is a large associated phlegmon, as well as diffuse peritonitis with rebound and guarding if free intra-abdominal perforation is present.

Diagnosis

The diagnosis of diverticulosis is based on patient history and clinical examination. Comprehensive diagnostic evaluation is recommended to confirm diverticulitis and help rule out other causes of abdominal pain. Laboratory findings in patients with diverticulitis may reveal leukocytosis and elevated C-reactive protein (CRP), however, these features are not specific for diverticulitis.[19] The diagnosis of diverticulitis made on clinical suspicion per clinical features and laboratory findings is correct in approximately 40% to 65% of patients.[20–22] Computed tomography (CT) imaging is therefore recommended to confirm the diagnosis of diverticulitis in patients without a prior imaging-confirmed diagnosis and to evaluate for potential complications in patients with severe presentations.[19] CT scan of the abdomen and pelvis with oral and intravenous contrast is highly accurate for diagnosing diverticulitis with sensitivity and specificity values of 95%.[21]

Treatment

The majority of patients with uncomplicated diverticulitis are managed in the outpatient setting with short-term diet modification, judicious analgesia, and antibiotics regimen if indicated. Multiple society guidelines currently recommend that antibiotics are not used routinely, but rather selectively in immunocompetent patients with acute uncomplicated diverticulitis cases.[19,23–25] Per the updated American Gastroenterology Association (AGA) guidelines, antibiotic treatment is advised in patients with acute uncomplicated diverticulitis who have multiple medical co-morbidities or frailty, refractory symptoms or vomiting, diverticulitis with fluid collection or longer segment of inflammation on CT scan, or who have CRP>140 mg/L or baseline leukocytosis >15 x 10^9 cells per liter.[19] Antibiotics should be tailored to gram-negative rods and anaerobes, most commonly metronidazole with a quinolone medication (eg, ciprofloxacin, levofloxacin) or trimethoprim/sulfamethoxazole, or amoxicillin/clavulanic acid monotherapy. A clear liquid diet is associated with symptomatic relief and is therefore typically advised on initial presentation for patient comfort,[26] and can be advanced as tolerated by the patient.

Treatment of complicated diverticulitis has a different approach and consists of broad-spectrum antibiotics and consultation with surgery for interventional source control management if indicated. This includes percutaneous drainage for significant pericolic abscesses or surgery for management of fistulas or strictures.

Gastroenterology Consultation/When to Refer

All patients with diverticulitis, including acute uncomplicated cases, are recommended for GI referral for colonoscopy evaluation after complete resolution of symptoms if a high-quality, updated colonoscopy is not performed within 1 year of the diverticulitis episode. A colonoscopy is typically recommended 6 to 8 weeks from onset of diverticulitis after symptom resolution, to confirm the presence of diverticula and to exclude any neoplasm or other colonic disease, as inflammatory bowel disease, that could mimic the symptoms of diverticulitis. An earlier colonoscopy may be considered if alarming symptoms are present.

Approximately 33% of patients after an initial episode of acute uncomplicated diverticulitis will have recurrent attacks or continue to have symptoms.[9] Additionally, a referral to colorectal surgery may be considered for patients with recurrent episodes of diverticulitis, as elective segmental colectomy reduces, but does not eliminate, diverticulitis risk.[27]

HEMORRHOIDS
Prevalence

The exact prevalence of symptomatic hemorrhoids is difficult to establish as it is underreported because patients do not seek care.[28] In 1989, the National Health Interview Survey reported that around 23 million adults (13% US population) were diagnosed with hemorrhoids in the prior year.[29] Unpublished data from the Healthcare Cost and Utilization Project on-line query system found 25,292 ambulatory surgery center visits for hemorrhoids and 203,552 Emergency Department visits in 2014 within 29 states. However, there are no national contemporary estimates of prevalence or health care costs related to hemorrhoids.[30]

Pathophysiology

Weakening of the submucosal connective cushion in the anal canal can cause downward displacement of the tissue producing venous dilation and prolapse. This is a multiple step process including (1) anchoring connective tissue deterioration; (2) prolapse of the hemorrhoidal tissue (3) abnormal distention of the arteriovenous anastomosis within the cushions; (4) abnormal dilation of the veins of the internal hemorrhoidal plexus.[16,31,32] Conditions causing increased venous pressure and altered venous drainage in the anal canal can precipitate hemorrhoid formation. These include

- Cirrhosis-ascites
- Pregnancy
- Frequent straining—prolonged standing or squatting
- Abnormal bowel function (diarrhea/constipation)
- Collagen vascular abnormalities
- Significant pelvic floor dysfunction
- Obesity
- Sedentarism

Recent studies showed matrix metalloproteinase (MMP) enzyme overexpressed in patients with hemorrhoids. MMP subtypes 9 and 2 are associated to break down

/degradation of proteins (elastin, fibronectin, collagen) of elastic fibers in the anal canal.[1] Other studies reported that endoglin (CD105), a proliferative marker for neovascularization, plays a role in the hemorrhoid formation.[33]

Clinical Presentation

Hemorrhoid symptoms vary with the extent of the disease process; some patients do not present symptoms.[34] Approximately 60% of the patients report hematochezia, 55% pruritus, 20% perianal discomfort, and 10% soiling.[35,36] *Non-painful* rectal bleeding typically associated with defecation is the cardinal symptom of internal hemorrhoids. Whereas external thrombosed hemorrhoids present with *painful* bleeding. Symptoms may be severe if there is increased venous pressure and altered venous drainage.

Prolapse is a sign used to classify the grade of internal hemorrhoids. Based on the extent of the protrusion, internal hemorrhoids are classified as grade 1 (there is no prolapse); grade 2 (prolapse with straining with spontaneous reduction post-defecation); grade 3 (prolapse and need for manual reduction); and grade 4 (prolapse not manually reducible) (**Fig. 3**).

Diagnosis

As part of a thorough history for hemorrhoids, it is important to ask about fiber and fluid intake, bowel patterns, bathroom habits (spending more than 3–4 minutes in the toilet

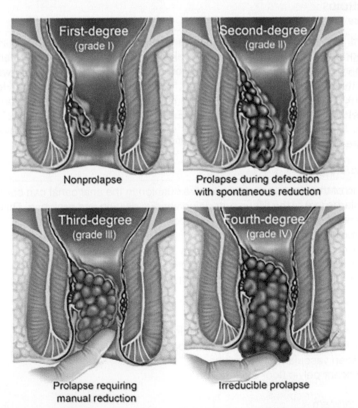

Fig. 3. Internal hemorrhoids grades. (*From* Lohsiriwat V. Chapter 5: Hemorrhoidal Disease. In: Coss-Adame E, Remes-Troche, JM, eds. Anorectal Disorders: Diagnosis and Non-Surgical Treatments. 1st ed. AP Press: 2019:51-63.)

may predispose to hemorrhoids formation), and the need for digital manipulation to aid in defecation.

The patient assessment should include digital examination and anoscopy in the left lateral or prone position. A digital rectal examination can detect masses, tenderness, and fluctuance. Internal hemorrhoids are unlikely to be palpable unless they are large or prolapsed.

Anoscopy is an effective way to visualize internal hemorrhoids. Physician should use terms relative to the patient to describe hemorrhoids' position (anterior, posterior, left, right) and avoid use of clockface terms.[37] Flexible endoscopy (sigmoidoscopy, colonoscopy) is not as accurate as anoscopy.[37] A study found that anoscopy identified 99% of anal lesions, whereas colonoscopy revealed only 78%.[38]

Treatment

Medical management: For symptomatic hemorrhoids, both internal and external conservative management includes

1. Increased fluid intake, 6 to 8 ounces/day
2. Increase dietary fiber intake 20 to 40 g/day or utilize fiber supplementation; fiber relieves symptoms and bleeding[31,39]
3. Encourage patients' use of sitz baths which lowers the sphincter and anal canal pressure[31]
4. Discourage increasing prolonged time on the toilet
5. Osmotic/stimulant laxatives and stool softeners if constipation is present despite increased fiber intake

Although nitroglycerin 0.4% ointment, topical nifedipine, and single botulin toxin injection into the anal sphincter canal are effective for pain relief,[40,41] there is not enough evidence to support the use of flavonoid supplements, topical anesthetic, keratolytic, protectants, and antiseptics. Hydrocortisone rectal cream or suppository is commonly prescribed as it provides both anti-inflammatory and analgesic effects, however, prolonged use of corticosteroids (no more than 1–2 weeks) is discouraged.[19,31]

Office-based procedures: Rubber band ligation (RBL) is a simple, low risk, recommended procedure to treat grade 1, 2, or 3 hemorrhoids and can be repeated in case of recurrence.[42,43] Complications (anorectal pain, bleeding, thrombosis of external hemorrhoids, and vasovagal symptoms) occurs only in 1% to 3% of patients. RBL should be used with caution in patients on anticoagulation.[42]

Sclerotherapy is reserved for hemorrhoids grade 1 or 2. It is useful for treating patients on anticoagulation and who are immunocompromised. RBL was reported superior to injection sclerotherapy to treat grades 1, 2 and 3 internal hemorrhoids.[31] Infrared coagulation (application of infrared heat via a device) is better suited for small to ligate bleeding type 1 or 2 hemorrhoids. Other treatment options in grades 1, 2 and 3 hemorrhoids are bipolar diathermy, direct current electrotherapy, and heater probe coagulation.

Thrombosed external hemorrhoids presenting with sudden onset of pain and swelling may be treated surgically if seen within 4 days.

Cryosurgery is no longer recommended in the United States because of postprocedure adverse effects: severe pain, discharge, and prolonged recovery.[14]

Surgical treatment: Nonsurgical approaches are successful in 80% to 99% of patients but sometimes advanced surgical interventions are indicated. Patients with grade 3 hemorrhoids unresponsive to nonsurgical approaches, grade 4 hemorrhoids, large external hemorrhoids, combined internal and external components and concomitant anorectal pathology are some indications for surgical interventions.[31] Classic closed hemorrhoidectomy is the most common technique in the United States and has been modified to include two alternative energy devices, Ligasure and Harmonic Scalpel. Hemorrhoidectomy is painful and associated with more blood loss and longer recovery time, but it has significantly lower rates of recurrence compared to office-based proced-ures.[31,43,45] Doppler-guided hemorrhoidal ligation with a hemorrhoidopexy, mucopexy, or a stapled hemorrhoidectomy; trans-anal hemorrhoidal dearterialization are newer surgical techniques. **Table 1** summarizes medical and procedural treatment options.

When to Refer

Noninvasive treatments for hemorrhoids can be applied by primary care doctors.[30] Patients with chronically bleeding grade 2 or 3 internal hemorrhoids unresponsive to conservative medical therapy should be referred to gastroenterology or colorectal sur-gery. Surgical referral is warranted in presence of refractory disease, patients who cannot tolerate office procedures, large external tags, large grades 3 and 4 internal hemorrhoids.[42]

ANORECTAL CONDITIONS
Prevalence

Anal fissures are common, with more than 200,000 new diagnoses occurring yearly in the United States.[46] In addition, the incidence of anal fissures is equal in male and fe-male patients and can impact all age groups.[46]

Low-risk HPV types 6 and 11 cause 90% of AGWs in patients.[47] However, HPV types 16, 18, 31,33, and 35 have been identified in AGWs despite being more commonly associated with malignancies.[2,47,48] Due to the high incidence and preva-lence of HPV, most sexually active people will be exposed to the virus in their life-time.[48] AGWs are common and widespread, a systematic review showed a global incidence in male and female patients ranging between 160 and 289 cases per 100,000.[49] In the United States, AGW incidence was estimated to be 1.2 cases per 1000 among women and 1.1 per 1000 cases among men.[48]

Previous studies of pruritis ani affect up to 5% of the population, however, most do not seek medical care as this can be a social embarrassing condition. It is more com-mon in men and in adults over the age of 30.[50]

Pathophysiology

An acute anal fissure is a superficial tear in the endoderm of the anal canal lasting less than 8 weeks.[42,51,52] A chronic anal fissure is a nonhealing ulcer that lasts greater than 8 weeks.[42] Increased pressure, often from the attempted passage of hard stools or repetitive trauma, can result in tears in the endoderm of the anal canal.[51] Due to the poor blood supply to the area, ischemia and decreased healing can occur in the area.[53] Anal fissures are often associated with a history of constipation, previous anal surgery, trauma, and a diet low in fiber which can result in hard stools.[51]

Human papillomavirus (HPV) is a double-stranded DNA virus that begins infection following disruption of the basal layer of the epithelium.[54] Anogenital HPV infections are transmitted through sexual contact via infected skin or mucosa.[55] Patients without clinical manifestations of HPV can spread the infection via sexual contact.[55] Notably, 90% of patients infected with a low- or high-risk HPV infection will clear the virus in 1 to 2 years without any clinical manifestations.[54]

The etiology of pruritis ani can vary, and a majority of cases are secondary to inflam-mation, infections, systemic disease, neoplasm, or an anorectal condition that causes the development of pruritis. **Table 2** summarizes common conditions causing perianal itching.

Table 1
Treatment options for internal hemorrhoids by grade

	Internal Hemorrhoids Grades				External	Mixed External Internal	Comments
	1	2	3	4			
Medical management	X	X	X	X	X	X	Modify fiber, fluid intake; sit baths, stool softeners, laxatives. Short course steroids
RBL	X	X	X				Low-risk, 1st line therapy, recommended by AGA
Sclerotherapy	X	X					Use in immunocompromised and patients on anticoagulation
Heater probe coagulation	X	X					Fast results, painful procedure
Infrared coagulation	X	X					Used in small to ligate hemorrhoids. High risk of recurrence
Bipolar diathermia	X	X	X				
Surgical treatment hemorrhoidectomy	(X)	(X)	X	X	X	X	If recurrence/resistance
							External thrombosed hemorrhoids should incised/excised within 4 days from symptoms onset

From Ganz RA. The evaluation and treatment of hemorrhoids: a guide for the gastroenterologist. Clin Gastroenterol Hepatol. 2013;11(6):593-603.

Table 2 Common conditions associated with pruritis ani	
Category	**Conditions**
Dermatologic	Inverse psoriasis Contact dermatitis Atopic dermatitis Hidradenitis suppurativa Bowen's disease (cutaneous squamous cell carcinoma in situ) Lichen planus
Anorectal disease	Internal hemorrhoids Abscesses Fissures Fistulas Constipation
Infection	Condyloma Herpes Syphilis Gonorrhea *Candida* *Enterobius vermicularis* (pinworm) Perianal streptococcal dermatitis Erythrasma (*Corynebacterium minutissimum*)
Systemic	Diabetes Cholestasis Lymphoma Leukemia Pellagra Renal failure Thyroid disease HIV disease Vitamins A, D, iron deficiencies
Diet/Medications*	Foods: coffee, tomatoes, beer, cola, tea, peanuts, milk products, citrus, chocolate, grapes Medications: tetracycline, colchicine, quinidine, peppermint oil, local anesthetics, neomycin
Fecal soilage	Diarrhea Abnormal recto-anal inhibitory reflex Internal anal sphincter relaxations abnormality

* May be direct irritants or cause irritation by causing loose stools or fecal seepage.

Clinical Presentation

Acute anal fissures appear to be a simple tear in the anal canal.[42] Chronic anal fissures may also have accompanying edema or fibrosis of the internal anal sphincter.[42] The location of the tear is inferior to the dentate line, with 90% of cases occurring along the posterior midline, where mucosal blood flow perfusion is significantly less than other quadrants.[42,51] Lateral anal fissures are atypical and may be secondary to other disease processes such as human immunodeficiency virus (HIV), Crohn's disease, and other granulomatous diseases (eg, TB, sarcoidosis).[42] Patients will present with a complaint of intense pain during and after stooling, potentially with a small amount of rectal bleeding.[51] In pruritis ani, the first symptom is often anal itching, but can also include perianal discomfort or skin lesions around the anal area.

For many patients, AGWs are asymptomatic and can go unnoticed. If symptomatic, patients may complain of an itching, painful, or burning sensation.[56] In addition, the presence of the lesions can be distressing to patients. The appearance of the warts is typically flat, papular, or pedunculated growths involving multiple areas of the anogenital region, including the perianal skin and anus.[47] The color of the warts is typically flesh-colored but can also range from white to brown.[3]

Diagnosis

Diagnosis of AGWs is usually made during the physical exam, and testing for HPV types is not recommended.[48] It is essential to keep in mind similar presenting conditions. The differential diagnosis of AGWs can include normal skin variations to other infectious causes such as condyloma lata caused by syphilis.[3] Therefore, if lesions are atypical (eg, pigmented, bleeding, ulcerated), the diagnosis is unclear; a biopsy should be considered, especially in immunocompromised patients.[2,47] Lesions that also fail to respond to standard therapies should also prompt consideration for a biopsy. Finally, patients with identified perianal or external anal warts should have their anal canal inspected via digital rectal exam or anoscopy for intra-anal lesions.[47]

A diagnosis of anal fissures is made on a physical examination. On visual examination, a simple tear may be seen; however, a chronic anal fissure may also be characterized by edema, fibrosis, and exposure of the muscular fibers of the internal anal sphincter.[42,46]

History for pruritis ani should include duration of symptoms, presence of generalized pruritis, association of itching with bowel movements, fecal seepage, systemic symptoms, history of other systemic illnesses, changes in diet or medications, anal hygiene practices, and tight fitting garment use.

A focused physical exam including digital exam of the anorectum should be performed to identify any anorectal or dermatological disease. Physical examination can be normal in appearance or slow maceration and super infection, with signs of lichenification of perianal skin resulting from chronic presentation.

Laboratory testing is generally not recommended to diagnose pruritis ani unless symptoms are refractory to management or there is concern for systemic disease. For these cases, the following testing can be considered.

- Complete blood count with differential to evaluate for evidence of malignancy, myeloproliferative disease, or iron deficiency
- Serum bilirubin, transaminases and alkaline phosphatase to evaluate for evidence of liver disease
- Thyroid-stimulating hormone to evaluate for evidence of a thyroid disorder
- Blood urea nitrogen and creatinine to evaluate for renal disease
- HIV antibody test in patients with risk factors for HIV infection

Treatment

In symptomatic patients, various treatment options are available to eliminate warts and improve symptoms.[2,47] In immunocompetent patients, warts can resolve spontaneously within 12 to 24 months.[55,56] Treatment should be guided based on the wart size, the amount, location of the lesion(s), and patient preference. Surgical interventions are more effective at wart removal when compared to topical medications but have a higher rate of occurrence; however, patient preference has historically been to initiate treatment with topical medication.[3,55] **Table 3** summarizes treatment options.

AGWs typically respond within the first 3 months of treatment; however, as the warts are sexually transmitted, recurrence can occur.[47] Patients with an identified AGW showed be screened and treated for co-current sexually transmitted infections.[56]

Table 3
Treatment options for anal warts

Drug	Patient or Provider Applied	Dosing/Route	Wart Location	Treatment Length	Side Effects
Imiquimod 3.75% cream	Patient	Topically applied once at bedtime every night	Use for external anal and perianal warts, not for intra-anal use	8 wks	Redness, irritation, and hypopigmentation *might weaken condoms and vaginal diaphragms*
Imiquimod 5% cream	Patient	Topically applied once at bedtime, 3x a week	Use for external anal and perianal warts, not for intra-anal use	16 wks	Redness, irritation, and hypopigmentation *might weaken condoms and vaginal diaphragms*
Podofilox 0.5% solution or gel	Patient	Topically applied 2x/day for 3 days, followed by 4 days of no therapy	Use for the external anus and perianal, not for intra-anal use—limit of <10 cm of skin	The treatment cycle can be repeated for up to four cycles	Redness, irritation, burning, inflammation.
Sinecatechins 15% ointment	Patient	Topically applied 3x/day	Use for the external anal and perianal warts, not for intra-anal use	It should be discontinued after 16 wks of use	Redness, itching/ burning pain, rash. Genital, anal, and oral sexual contact should be avoided and not recommended for patients with HIV or other immunocompromised conditions.

Cryotherapy	Provider	Once per week, application of liquid nitrogen by a trained provider	It can be used in external, perianal, and intra-anal warts		Pain during and after application of liquid nitrogen. It can lead to scarring and inflammation.
Surgical Removal	Provider	Anesthesia then removal of warts by a trained provider	It can be used in external, perianal, and intra-anal warts	Able to eliminate all/majority of warts in a single visit	Scarring. Post-operative pain. Possible need for general anesthesia. Treatment of warts should be performed in a well-ventilated room following standard precautions.
Trichloroacetic acid (TCA)	Provider	Once per week	It can be used in external, perianal, and intra-anal warts	Can be repeated weekly	Pain, ulceration.
Bichloroacetic Acid (BCA) 80%–90% solution	Provider	Once per week	It can be used in external, perianal, and intra-anal warts	Can be repeated weekly	Pain, ulceration.

However, if a patient fails to respond to the initial patient or provider applied treatment, an alternative medication/procedure should be initiated.

Prevention in the form of vaccination is an essential step in stopping the spread of anal warts. The Advisory Committee on Immunization Practices recommends the HPV vaccination series as a part of the standard childhood vaccination schedule until 26 years of age.[47] Shared decision-making between patients and physicians about proceeding with the vaccine after age 26 should be considered in special populations.[47] To be effective, vaccinations should be provided before possible virus exposure.

Conservative measures are the first-line treatment of acute anal fissures. Management should focus on softening stools, ensuring easier stool passage, and increasing dietary fiber intake and fluid intake to prevent the reoccurrence of anal fissures.[51,57,58] Close to 50% of acute anal fissures will heal with a combination of sitz baths and increased fiber supplementation.[42] However, if the patient is still symptomatic, topical analgesics and vasodilators should be considered for therapy. A combination of topical lidocaine gel and stool softeners has an estimated heal rate of 16% to 31% in both acute and chronic fissures.[57] **Table 4** summarizes treatment options for acute anal fissures.

Medical management is the first-line treatment of chronic anal fissures but may also require surgical management if conservative measures fail. Topical calcium channel blockers are the first line in treating chronic anal fissures.[42] **Table 5** summarizes treatment options for chronic anal fissures.

Initial treatment of pruritis ani consists of treating the presumed underlying cause. This includes improving anal hygiene, avoiding moisture in the anal area, removing offending medications or foods from the diet, and adequate skin protection.

In refractory cases that do not resolve with initial treatment measures, one should consider laboratory analysis (see Diagnosis section) and full thickness punch biopsy. If no etiology is found, consider topical capsaicin (three times per day for 4 weeks) or anal tattooing with methylene blue, though there is limited evidence to support these treatment options.[60–62]

When to Refer

Although treatment of AGWs is within the scope of practice for the primary care physician, there are select reasons to initiate a referral to gastroenterology. The presence of intra-anal lesions should prompt a referral to gastroenterology/colorectal for further evaluation and management.[47] Patients with warts that are too large for topical medications or cryotherapy should be referred.[3] In addition, a referral to a specialist is recommended if the patient's disease is refractory to multiple rounds of treatment or if there is a concern for outlet obstruction involving the anus.[3]

Table 4
Treatment options for acute anal fissures

Medication	Dose	Route
Sitz bath	10–15 min of immersion two to three times daily	Topical
Fiber[58]	18–30 g per day	PO
Stool softeners	Various	PO
Lidocaine gel[53]	2% gel to be placed three times daily for 14 d maximum	Topical
Nitrates	0.2% or 0.4% ointment twice daily for 8 wks	Topical
Nifedipine	0.2%–0.3% ointment used two to four times daily	Topical

Table 5
Treatment options for chronic anal fissures

Medication	Dose	Route	Side Effects	Efficacy
Nitrates	0.1%, 0.2%, or 0.4% twice a day for 8 wks	Topical	Headaches	36%–57%
Calcium Channel Blockers	Nifedipine: 0.2%–0.5% ointment twice daily for 8 weeks	Topical	Nifedipine: Headaches	67%–90%
• Nifedipine				
• Diltiazem[59]	Diltiazem: 2% rectal gel three times daily for 8 wks			
Botulinum toxin A[46]	Max of two injections	Injection	Fecal incontinence	60%–80%
Lateral internal sphincterotomy[46]	N/A	Surgical	Risk associated with general anesthesia	85%
			Fecal incontinence	

For anal fissures, referral to a specialist in colorectal disease should be considered in patients with persistent pain after 8 weeks or if the fissure is still present after 16 weeks, with or without pain.[58] If the anal fissure is secondary to a condition such as HIV, tuberculosis, Crohn's disease, or ulcerative colitis, it should prompt a referral to the appropriate specialists.[51,58]

Pruritis ani should be referred out in refractory cases to rule out other potential etiologies and for other treatment options.

SUMMARY

Benign conditions of the lower GI tract are very common and the role of the primary care physician in the initial workup and management is well-recognized. A majority of the conditions reviewed above can be managed in the outpatient setting by the primary care physician. Like most health conditions, the key to diagnosis is a through history and focused physical exam based on clinical symptoms. Diverticular diseases, including diverticulitis, continue to rise among adults in the United States. Judicious use of antibiotics in mild cases is now recommended. Surveillance and monitoring of diverticular disease by colorectal disease specialists is recommended. Hemorrhoids affect almost 5% of the US population, and conservative management is recommended in most cases. RBL is the recommended first-line treatment of internal hemorrhoids. Anogenital warts are most commonly causes by HPV strains 6 and 11, which may be prevented with early childhood vaccinations. Anal fissures can become a chronic and painful condition for some; treatment options include topicals. Pruritis ani is likely underreported. This condition is generally secondary to another underlying condition, thus, a thorough history and physical is essential for guidance of treatment.

CLINICS CARE POINTS

- Diverticulosis, defined by the presence of diverticula, is largely asymptomatic but can be associated with bleeding, infection, perforation, fistula, or obstruction.
- Selected patients with uncomplicated diverticulitis may be treated conservatively without antibiotics.
- Painless bleeding and intermittent protrusion are the main presenting symptoms of hemorrhoids.
- Internal hemorrhoids are classified on grade 1 (do not prolapse); grade 2 (prolapse but spontaneously reduce); grade 3 (prolapse and require manual reduction); and grade 4 (protrude and cannot be reduced).
- Medical conservative management is the recommended initial treatment in symptomatic grades 1, 2, and 3 internal and external hemorrhoids.
- Acute thrombosed hemorrhoids should be managed with surgical excision within the first 4 days of onset of symptoms.
- About 90% of anogenital warts are caused by HPV type 6 and 11 and spread via direct contact with infected skin/mucosa.
- Anal fissures are superficial tears in the anal canal and can cause a significant amount of pain.
- Chronic anal fissures' first-line management includes topical calcium channel blockers but may require surgical interventions if conservative measures fail.
- Pruritis ani is a common yet underreported condition that is generally secondary to another underlying etiology.

DISCLOSURE

The authors have nothing to disclose.

FUNDING

MKS is supported in part by NIMHD K23 MD015088-04 and Emory School of Medicine Doris Duke Charitable Foundation COVID-19 Fund to Retain Clinical Scientists and the Georgia CTSA (UL1-TR002378).

REFERENCES

1. Lohsiriwat V. Hemorrhoids: from basic pathophysiology to clinical management. WJG 2009;18(17). https://doi.org/10.3748/wjg.v18.i17.2009.
2. Buck H. Warts (genital). BMJ Clin Evid 2010;2010:1602.
3. O'Mahony C, Gomberg M, Skerlev M, et al. Position statement for the diagnosis and management of anogenital warts. J Eur Acad Dermatol Venereol JEADV 2019;33(6):1006–19.
4. Kaise M, Nagata N, Ishii N, et al. Epidemiology of colonic diverticula and recent advances in the management of colonic diverticular bleeding. Dig Endosc 2020; 32(2):240–50.
5. Everhart JE, Ruhl CE. Burden of digestive diseases in the United States part II: lower gastrointestinal diseases. Gastroenterology 2009;136(3):741–54.
6. Strate LL, Modi R, Cohen E, et al. Diverticular disease as a chronic illness: evolving epidemiologic and clinical insights. Am J Gastroenterol 2012;107(10): 1486–93.
7. SHAHEDI K, FULLER G, BOLUS R, et al. Long-term Risk of Acute Diverticulitis Among Patients With Incidental Diverticulosis Found During Colonoscopy. Clin Gastroenterol Hepatol 2013;11(12):1609–13.
8. Bharucha AE, Parthasarathy G, Ditah I, et al. Temporal Trends in the Incidence and Natural History of Diverticulitis: A Population-Based Study. Am J Gastroenterol 2015;110(11):1589–96.
9. Sabiston Textbook of surgery - 21st ed. Published August 10, 2022. https://www.clsevier.com/books/sabiston-textbook-of-surgery/townsend/978-0-323-64062-6. Accessed 9 August, 2022.
10. Aldoori WH, Giovannucci EL, Rimm EB, et al. A prospective study of diet and the risk of symptomatic diverticular disease in men. Am J Clin Nutr 1994;60(5): 757–64.
11. Aldoori WH, Giovannucci EL, Rimm EB, et al. Prospective study of physical activity and the risk of symptomatic diverticular disease in men. Gut 1995;36(2): 276–82.
12. Strate LL, Liu YL, Aldoori WH, et al. Obesity increases the risks of diverticulitis and diverticular bleeding. Gastroenterology 2009;136(1):115–22.e1.
13. Hjern F, Wolk A, Håkansson N. Smoking and the risk of diverticular disease in women. Br J Surg 2011;98(7):997–1002.
14. Strate LL, Keeley BR, Cao Y, et al. Western Dietary Pattern Increases, and Prudent Dietary Pattern Decreases, Risk of Incident Diverticulitis in a Prospective Cohort Study. Gastroenterology 2017;152(5):1023–30.e2.
15. Strate LL, Liu YL, Syngal S, et al. Nut, corn, and popcorn consumption and the incidence of diverticular disease. JAMA 2008;300(8):907–14.
16. Camilleri M, Sandler RS, Peery AF. Etiopathogenetic mechanisms in diverticular disease of the colon. Cell Mol Gastroenterol Hepatol 2019;9(1):15–32.

17. Boostrom SY, Wolff BG, Cima RR, et al. Uncomplicated diverticulitis, more complicated than we thought. J Gastrointest Surg 2012;16(9):1744–9.
18. Kaiser AM, Jiang JK, Lake JP, et al. The management of complicated diverticulitis and the role of computed tomography. Am J Gastroenterol 2005;100(4):910–7.
19. Peery AF, Shaukat A, Strate LL. AGA Clinical Practice Update on Medical Management of Colonic Diverticulitis: Expert Review. Gastroenterology 2021;160(3): 906–11.e1.
20. Andeweg CS, Knobben L, Hendriks JCM, et al. How to diagnose acute left-sided colonic diverticulitis: proposal for a clinical scoring system. Ann Surg 2011; 253(5):940–6.
21. Laméris W, van Randen A, Bipat S, et al. Graded compression ultrasonography and computed tomography in acute colonic diverticulitis: Meta-analysis of test accuracy. Eur Radiol 2008;18(11):2498–511.
22. Laméris W, van Randen A, van Gulik TM, et al. A clinical decision rule to establish the diagnosis of acute diverticulitis at the emergency department. Dis Colon Rectum 2010;53(6):896–904.
23. Hall J, Hardiman K, Lee S, et al. The American Society of Colon and Rectal Surgeons Clinical Practice Guidelines for the Treatment of Left-Sided Colonic Diverticulitis. Dis Colon Rectum 2020;63(6):728–47.
24. Sartelli M, Weber DG, Kluger Y, et al. 2020 update of the WSES guidelines for the management of acute colonic diverticulitis in the emergency setting. World J Emerg Surg 2020;15(1):32.
25. Francis NK, Sylla P, Abou-Khalil M, et al. EAES and SAGES 2018 consensus conference on acute diverticulitis management: evidence-based recommendations for clinical practice. Surg Endosc 2019;33(9):2726–41.
26. Stam MaW, Draaisma WA, van de Wall BJM, et al. An unrestricted diet for uncomplicated diverticulitis is safe: results of a prospective diverticulitis diet study. Colorectal Dis 2017;19(4):372–7.
27. Thornblade LW, Simianu VV, Davidson GH, et al. Elective Surgery for Diverticulitis and the Risk of Recurrence and Ostomy. Ann Surg 2021;273(6):1157–64.
28. Madoff R, Fleshman J. American Gastroenterological Association technical review on the diagnosis and treatment of hemorrhoids. Gastroenterology 2004; 126(5):1463–73.
29. Le Clere FB, Moss AJ, Everhart JA, et al. Prevalence of major digestive disorders and bowel symptoms, 1989. Adv Data 1992;24(212):1–15.
30. Sandlers R, Peery A. Rethinking What We Know About Hemorrhoids. Clin Gastroenterol Hepatol 2019;17(1):8–15.
31. Ganz R. The Evaluation and Treatment of Hemorrhoids. A Guide for the Gastroenterologist 2013;11:593–603.
32. Thomson WH. The nature of haemorrhoids. BJG. 18(17. Br J Surg 1975;62: 542–52.
33. Chung Y. Endoglin (CD105) expression in the development of hemorrhoids. Eur J Investig 2004;34(2):107–12.
34. Riss S, Weiser F, Schwameis K, et al. The prevalence of hemorrhoids in adults. Int J Colorectal Dis 2012;27:215–20.
35. Mott T, Lattimer K, Edwards C. Hemorrhoids: Diagnosis and Treatment Options. Am Fam Med 2018;97(3):172–9.
36. Jacobs D. Hemorrhoids. N Engl J Med 2014;371:944–51.
37. Guttenplan M. The Evaluation and Office Management of Hemorrhoids for the Gastroenterologist. Curr Gastroenterol Rep 2017;19(7):30.

38. Kelly S, Sanowski R, Foutch P, et al. A prospective comparison of anoscopy and fiberendoscopy in detecting anal lesions. J Clin Gastroenterol 1986;8(6):658–60.

39. Alonso-Coello P, Guyatt G, Heels-Ansdell D, et al. Laxatives for the treatment of hemorrhoids. Cochrane Database of Systematic Reviews 2005. https://doi.org/10.1002/14651858.CD004649.pub2.

40. Perrotti P, Antropoli C, Molino D, et al. Conservative treatment of acute thrombosed external hemorrhoids with topical nifedipine. Dis Colon Rectum 2001; 44(3):405–9.

41. Patti R, Arcara M, Bonventre S, et al. Randomized clinical trial of botulinum toxin injection for pain relief in patients with thrombosed external haemorrhoids. Br J Surg 2008;95(11):1339–43.

42. Wald Λ, Bharucha A, Limketkai B, et al. ACG Clinical Guidelines: Management of Benign Anorectal Disorders. Am J Gastroenterol 2021;116:1987–2008.

43. McRae M, McLeod S. Comparison of hemorrhoidal treatment modalities. A meta-analysis. Dis Colon Rectum 1995;38(7):687–94.

44. Kaidar-Person O, Person B, Wexner S. Hemorrhoidal disease: A comprehensive review. J Am Coll Surg 2007;204(1):102–17.

45. Jutabha R, Jensen D, Chavalitdhamrong D. Randomized prospective study of endoscopic rubber band ligation compared with bipolar coagulation for chronically bleeding internal hemorrhoids. Am J Gastroenterol 2009;104(8):2057–64.

46. Madalinski MH. Identifying the best therapy for chronic anal fissure. World J Gastrointest Pharmacol Ther 2011;2(2):9–16.

47. Centers for Disease Control and Prevention. Anogenital Warts 2021.

48. Park IU, Introcaso C, Dunne EF. Human Papillomavirus and Genital Warts: A Review of the Evidence for the 2015 Centers for Disease Control and Prevention Sexually Transmitted Diseases Treatment Guidelines. Clin Infect Dis Off Publ Infect Dis Soc Am 2015;61(Suppl 8):S849–55.

49. Patel H, Wagner M, Singhal P, et al. Systematic review of the incidence and prevalence of genital warts. BMC Infect Dis 2013;13:39.

50. Siddiqi S, Vijay V, Ward M, et al. Pruritus Ani. Ann R Coll Surg Engl 2008;90(6): 457–63.

51. Jahnny B, Ashurst JV. Anal fissures. Treasure Island, FL: StatPearls Publishing; 2023.

52. Stewart DB, Gaertner W, Glasgow S, et al. Clinical Practice Guideline for the Management of Anal Fissures. Dis Colon Rectum 2017;60(1):7–14.

53. Kujur ADS, Paul Ekka NM, Chandra S, et al. Comparative Study to Assess the Effectiveness of Topical Nifedipine and Diltiazem in the Treatment of Chronic Anal Fissure. J Fam Med Prim Care 2020;9(11):5652–7.

54. de Sanjosé S, Brotons M, Pavón MA. The natural history of human papillomavirus infection. Best Pract Res Clin Obstet Gynaecol 2018;47:2–13.

55. Leslie SW, Sajjad H, Kumar S. Genital warts. Treasure Island, FL: StatPearls Publishing; 2023. Available at: https://www.ncbi.nlm.nih.gov/books/NBK441884/.

56. Lopaschuk CC. New approach to managing genital warts. Can Fam Physician Med Fam Can 2013;59(7):731–6.

57. Gardner IH, Siddharthan RV, Tsikitis VL. Benign anorectal disease: hemorrhoids, fissures, and fistulas. Ann Gastroenterol 2020;33(1):9–18.

58. Newman M, Collie M. Anal fissure: diagnosis, management, and referral in primary care. Br J Gen Pract J R Coll Gen Pract 2019;69(685):409–10.

59. Knight JS, Birks M, Farouk R. Topical diltiazem ointment in the treatment of chronic anal fissure. Br J Surg 2001;88(4):553–6.

60. Farouk R, Lee PW. Intradermal methylene blue injection for the treatment of intractable idiopathic pruritus ani. Br J Surg 1997;84(5):670.
61. Mentes BB, Akin M, Leventoglu S, et al. Intradermal methylene blue injection for the treatment of intractable idiopathic pruritus ani: results of 30 cases. Tech Coloproctology 2004;8(1):11–4.
62. Eusebio EB, Graham J, Mody N. Treatment of intractable pruritus ani. Dis Colon Rectum 1990;33(9):770–2.

Colorectal Cancer Screening and Iron Deficiency Anemia

Ethan P. Berg, DO[a,b], Asiya Mohammed, MD[b,c], Zachary J. Shipp, MD, MS[a,b], Johnny C. Tenegra, MD, MS[a,b,d],*

KEYWORDS

- Colorectal cancer screening • Colon cancer • Screening guidelines
- Iron deficiency anemia • Iron supplementation

KEY POINTS

- Screening in adults for colorectal cancer should start at 45 years of age according to multiple governing medical bodies. This can be achieved with either direct visualization or stool-based testing.
- Iron deficiency anemia can be diagnosed most accurately with a ferritin count.
- Both oral and parenteral therapy can be used to treat iron deficiency anemia, but parenteral therapy is not shown to have significantly higher risk for serious adverse advents as previously thought.

COLORECTAL CANCER SCREENING
Introduction

Comparing the average number of annual new cancer cases in the United States from 2014 to 2018, colorectal cancer (CRC) ranked fourth[1] with 142,462 new CRC cases reported.[2] Many cases are due to sporadic mutations or DNA mismatch repair.[3] Males had a higher rate of having and dying from CRC compared with females. Five-year relative survival for colon cancer was highest at 88% when found at a localized stage, dropping to 16% when diagnosed at a distant stage. According to the Centers for Disease Control and Prevention, 71.6% of adults who were aged 50 to 75 years were up-to-date on colorectal screening.[4] The rate of colon cancer, in people over the age of 50 years has been steadily declining between 2014 and 2018 by roughly 2% per year, although there has been a commensurate increase in the cancer rate in those less

[a] SIU Decatur Family Medicine Residency, 102 West Kenwood Avenue, Ste 100, Decatur, IL 62526, USA; [b] Department of Family & Community Medicine, Southern Illinois University School of Medicine, Springfield, IL, USA; [c] SIU Springfield Family Medicine Residency, 520 N. 4th Street, Springfield, IL 62702, USA; [d] Department of Family & Community Medicine, Southern Illinois University School of Medicine Decatur Family Medicine Residency, Decatur, IL, USA
* Corresponding author.
E-mail address: jtenegra@siumed.edu

Prim Care Clin Office Pract 50 (2023) 481–491
https://doi.org/10.1016/j.pop.2023.03.008
0095-4543/23/© 2023 Elsevier Inc. All rights reserved.
primarycare.theclinics.com

than 50 years old.[5] Most CRC develops spontaneously from adenomatous polyps, whereas a minority develops from sessile serrated lesions.[6]

SCREENING/DIAGNOSIS
Recommendations and Guidelines

Several screening guidelines by various medical societies have been published with similar but slightly variable recommendations. A brief summary of these screening recommendations is listed in **Table 1**.[7–9] For those with one or more first-degree relatives with a history of CRC, cancer screening should start at either age 40 or 10 years before the age of the youngest diagnosed family member, whichever is earlier. The US Preventative Services Task Force (USPSTF) recommendations include several options for screening strategies. It does not make a recommendation as to which is the best strategy to use, but considerations can be made for factors beyond the accuracy of the tests. For example, patient acceptance/compliance, risks/benefits, and cost-effectiveness may all be considered. Individual factors that may influence a given patient's compliance include cost out of pocket, time off from work, patient concerns of endoscopy, ability or comfort to self-collect a stool sample, or frequency of testing. Patients may also have concerns regarding endoscopy, such as bowel preparation or concerns about camera insertion. The approved screening strategies can generally be divided into direct visualization testing and indirect testing, which includes computed tomography (CT) colonography and stool-based testing.

Direct Visualization Techniques

Colonoscopy should be performed whenever another CRC screening test is positive. However, colonoscopy can be also used as primary screening. Colonoscopy, such as flexible sigmoidoscopy, gives direct visualization of the colon. Flexible sigmoidoscopy visualizes only the terminal 50 cm of the colon, whereas colonoscopy covers the entire colon up to the terminal ileum. Patients are given a purgative agent for preparation and are typically sedated for a colonoscopy but not for sigmoidoscopy. Currently, no randomized clinical control trial has been completed to evaluate the efficacy of colonoscopy. There is a current randomized trial underway called the Nordic-European Initiative on Colorectal Cancer, which aims to compare colonoscopy to no organized screen with regard to incidence and mortality.[10]

Flexible sigmoidoscopy gives direct visualization of the distal colorectum and allows for biopsy and removal of colon polyps. Patients are given bowel preparation with enemas with or without the addition of magnesium citrate. The procedure is performed without sedation. Four long-term randomized control trials have looked at the efficacy of flexible sigmoidoscopy compared with no screening. One of these studies found that one flexible sigmoidoscopy provided the reduced risk of diagnosis and death from CRC for at least 17 years.[11] Two of the studies found a reduction in incidence and mortality of CRC.[12,13] The final study found reduced incidence and mortality in men but found little to no effect in women.[14] This difference was explained largely by the fact women are more likely than men to develop more proximal cancers. The protocol for a flexible sigmoidoscopy with abnormal findings is to follow with a colonoscopy to visualize the remainder of the colon.

Indirect Testing

CT colonography

CT colonography (CTC) as a screen is performed every 5 years. It involves first completing a bowel preparation regimen similar to a colonoscopy and restricting diet to clear liquids the day before the examination. During the examination, the distal colon

Table 1
Recommendations for colorectal cancer screening, asymptomatic adults at average risk

Organization	Screening Test and Recommended Screening Interval	Patient Age
US Preventive Services Task Force[6]	High-sensitivity guaiac fecal occult blood test (gFOBT) or fecal immunochemical test (FIT)—1 y Stool DNA-FIT—1–3 y CT colonography, 5 y Flexible sigmoidoscopy, 5 y Flexible sigmcidoscopy + annual FIT, 10 y Colonoscopy, 10 y	Screen adults aged 45–49 y. Screen all adults aged 50–75 y.
American College of Gastroenterology[7]	Colonoscopy, 10 y Flexible sigmoidoscopy, 5–10 y CT colonography, 5 y Colon video capsule 5 y FITs , 1 y Multi-target DNA stool test (mt-sDNA), 3 years	Start colorectal cancer screening at 50 y of age, but offer it at 45 y of age for average-risk patients.
American Cancer Society[8]	FITs, 1 y and gFOBT, 1 y mt-sDNA, 3 y Flexible sigmoidoscopy, 5 y CT colonography, 5 y Colonoscopy, 10 y	People at average risk of colorectal cancer screening, should start at 45 y of age, and screen until 75 y of age.

and rectum are insufflated, and a low-dose CT scan, which does not require IV contrast agent, is performed. It is faster and less invasive than a colonoscopy, and there is less chance of a bowel perforation. Also, unlike a colonoscopy, CTC does not require sedation and its associated risk. These may be relevant considerations for patients with a history of breathing problems, who are on blood thinners, or for those with an abdominal surgical history. However, the potential downsides include a relatively higher cost than the fecal screening tests, radiation exposure from the scanner, and suboptimal result interpretation, which depends on a trained radiologist. One unique risk to CTC is the potential for incidental findings on the image that may require their own follow-up independent of considerations for colonic findings. A positive colonic finding would require a follow-up colonoscopy. A meta-analysis of randomized-control trials comparing CTC with colonoscopy in average-risk adults showed that although it has greater than 90% sensitivity for detecting adenomatous and serrated polyps of greater than 10 mm, it is less sensitive for flat or sessile polyps.[15]

Guaiac Fecal Occult Blood Test

Guaiac fecal occult blood test (gFOBT) is an annual testing strategy that requires collection of multiple stool samples by the patient in their home, which are then tested for the presence of occult blood using a chemical indicator. It generally has the lowest cost per test among the commonly used screening strategies but is conducted more frequently (annually). Historically, there were dietary and medication restrictions such as reducing red meat, iron supplements, NSAIDs, and high-vitamin C-containing foods in the days preceding the testing, but this was found to not significantly impact testing specificity and has been abandoned as a recommendation.[16] There are no potential safety or concerns for harm beyond those associated with follow-up colonoscopies if indicated. A positive screen would require such a follow-up colonoscopy. Based on five randomized control trials on intention to screen basis, screening with gFOBT testing was associated with reduced CRC mortality compared with no screening after two to nine rounds of screening at up to 30 years of follow-up (relative risk [RR], 0.91 [95% confidence interval (CI), 0.84–0.98] at 19.5 years.[17]

Fecal Immunochemical Testing (FIT)

Fecal immunochemical testing (FIT) is an annual testing strategy similar to gFOBT wherein a stool sample collected by the patient in their own home can be directly assayed for occult blood. Unlike gFOBT, however, the detection uses an antibody directed against human hemoglobin rather than a chemical indicator which changes color in the presence of blood AND only requires a single stool sample. It is more specific than gFOBT testing as it should only indicate the presence of blood coming from the colon where the hemoglobin has not yet had time to degrade in the upper gastrointestinal tract. Like gFOBT testing, there are no direct risks or danger of harm from this testing. A positive screen would necessitate a follow-up colonoscopy. One large (n~5,420,000) prospective national study conducted in Taiwan examined the relationship between FIT testing and CRC mortality. This study found that one to three rounds of screening with a biennial FIT test lowered CRC mortality at 6 years' follow-up, compared with no screening (adjusted RR, 0.90 [95%CI, 0.84–0.95]).[18]

Stool DNA–Fecal Immunochemical Testing(Cologuard)

Stool DNA-FIT (sDNA-FIT) testing is similar to classic FIT testing whereby it detects the presence of hemoglobin in the stool, but it additionally tests the stool for cells shed from the colon mucosa for 10 DNA biomarkers associated with CRC.[19] This increases the sensitivity for more proximal polyps, sessile serrated polys, and high-grade dysplasia relative to FIT testing alone, but also decreases the specificity for CRC from 95% for FIT to 87% for sDNA-FIT.[20] Similar to the other stool testing methods, the patient collects a sample in their home and then submits the testing kit by mail for analysis with no specific health risks. It is more expensive than FOBT or FIT testing. The testing is performed every 3 years, with a follow-up colonoscopy if it returns positive.

Emerging Screening Method

One novel strategy for detecting colon cancer which does not require procedural direct visualization or collecting a stool sample that has limited US Food and Drug Administration (FDA) approval is the methylated SEPT9 DNA plasma assay (Epi Pro-Colon). It is not included in the latest USPSTF recommended strategies due to insufficient supporting evidence, although research is ongoing. mSEPT9 DNA testing is a blood-based cancer screening strategy. Cytosine residues in the v2 promoter region of the SEPT9 gene may become hyper-methylated in CRC. The technique uses a chemical treatment to identify the methylated base pairs in the gene and then specific primers for RT-PCR to amplify and analyze the gene.[7]

In the prospective clinical trial (PRESEPT clinical trial) using PCR for amplification and detection of methylated SEPT9 DNA in blood of average risk adults (n = 1544), sensitivity for all stages of CRC was 68% (95% CI 53%-80%).[21] A single-arm longitudinal Prospective Cohort Post-Approval Study is ongoing at the FDA to evaluate the effectiveness of the Epi ProColon tests in adults over the age of 50 years at average risk for developing CRC and is scheduled to complete in early 2023.[22]

Need for Ongoing Research

Although the benefit of CRC screening in average-risk individuals is well established, there is an ongoing need for research into the effectiveness of the newer screening strategies as well as hybrid strategies where multiple modalities are used over time. It is of interest how the strategies' effectiveness may change over the lifespan given the increasing risk with age, whereas, there is a developing trend toward increasing prevalence of colon cancer in adults younger than 50 years old. The recommendations of the USPTF rely on compliance estimates of 100%, which may be impractical. Modeling that accounts for evolving testing accuracy, cancer prevalence rates, changing average lifespan, and effectiveness of interventions after diagnosis may ultimately identify a preferred strategy. Further, as health care spending continues to increase and care is thoughtfully rationed, it is important to study where the health care dollars may be most effectively spent.

Beyond optimizing the testing strategy, further research is also needed in regard to patient compliance with the recommendations. In the United States, prevalence among adults aged 50 to 75 years who reported being current with CRC screening recommendations has increased over the last decade to 71.8% (95% CI 71.2–72.4).[23] Studying colon cancer screening through the lens of the social determinants of health may allow for policy that increases screening participation and improved outcomes.

IRON DEFICIENCY ANEMIA
Introduction

Iron deficiency anemia (IDA) is thought to affect women of childbearing age most commonly. However, it can occur in any demographic of patients. Iron is a necessary element required for the transport of oxygen throughout the body for regulation of all cellular functions, and red blood cells serve to hold the iron needed for this function. Gastrointestinal causes represent a significant underlying etiology of IDA, ranging from issues related to intake, absorption, and gastrointestinal blood loss. Most significantly, cancer of the gastrointestinal tract can manifest in this way as well. It is imperative to note these causes when evaluating patients with anemia.

Anemia affected 40% of the world's children aged 6 to 59 months, 30% of nonpregnant women aged 15 to 49 years, 36% of pregnant women 15 to 49 years.[24] Men and postmenopausal women have lower rates of IDA, ranging from 2% to 5% in the United States, northern Europe, and Canada.[25] The difference in rates of anemia between men and women of childbearing age can be explained most commonly by menstruation, whereas children suffer from IDA most commonly because of inadequate dietary intake. In men and postmenopausal women, a gastrointestinal cause for anemia is most likely the cause. These statistics highlight the ubiquity of IDA, making it the most common nutritional disorder encountered by clinicians.

Pathophysiology

WHO has defined anemia as hemoglobin less than 130 g/L in men, less than 120 g/L in nonpregnant women, and less than 110 g/L in pregnant women.[26] Hepcidin is an important mediator of iron recycling and absorption and acts by blocking the action of ferroportin.[27] This results in a decreased release of iron into the plasma. During times of anemia, hepcidin is suppressed, which results in more iron being absorbed and recycled by dying red blood cells. In periods of inflammation, hepcidin is increased, which results in decreased iron and subsequent anemia. Erythropoietin is stimulated by hypoxia, which results in the release of red blood cells that do not have appropriate iron in the setting of anemia. As a result, hepcidin is further suppressed. In the setting of hypoxia, more iron is absorbed through the gut as well.

Intake and absorption of iron

Iron is ingested in food in two main forms: non-heme and heme iron. Non-heme iron is found in any source of plants, whereas heme iron is ingested through any form of animal meat. In an ideal diet, 5 to 15 mg of Fe, and 1 to 5 mg of heme iron are taken in daily. If there is inadequate intake, this can result in IDA and malnutrition can be considered the underlying cause.

The two forms of iron are absorbed differently in the gut, mainly at the duodenum and proximal jejunum. Numerous cotransporters assist with the breakdown and subsequent absorption, and genetic mutations of these can lead to problems with absorption. Inflammatory conditions of the gastrointestinal tract can also result in anemia, such as infection with *Helicobacter pylori* or celiac disease. Surgical removal of the absorptive areas of the gut, such as with gastric bypass surgery, can also lead to problems with absorption and require subsequent supplementation.

Certain dietary practices can also result in decreased absorption, such as with tea and coffee.[26] In addition, certain medications can also affect absorption such as proton-pump inhibitors. In all of these conditions, it may not suffice to supplement with iron, as the underlying issue is with absorption. In these instances, it is important to treat the underlying issue as opposed to increasing iron intake. In conditions that result in chronic inflammation, such as autoimmune diseases, chronic infections, or obesity, iron stores may not be properly mobilized. There are also conditions in which erythropoietin release is stimulated because of anemia. However, the anemia is not corrected because of limited iron stores.

Loss and increased demand

Blood loss of the gastrointestinal tract can also manifest as IDA. Erosive conditions, such as peptic ulcer disease, or bleeding cancerous masses lead to significant occult losses that are not always perceptible by patients. These losses can be slow and often symptoms do not manifest until a threshold has been crossed. Physiologically, menstruation can also result in chronic losses and result in IDA as well.[26] This also occurs in individuals who donate blood often as well as patients who are on dialysis. Infections with parasites or worms can lead to chronic blood loss through the gastrointestinal tract. Medications are implicated in this cause of anemia as well, such as with aspirin and steroids that lead to irritation of the lining of the gut. Infants, children, adolescents, and pregnancy represent times during which physiologically the body requires more iron. This can be exacerbated in developing countries due to malnutrition or diets that are low in iron.[26]

Clinical Presentation

Symptoms of IDA[28] are similar to that of other symptoms of anemia and may include.

- fatigue
- impaired exercise outcomes
- poor concentration
- dizziness
- tinnitus
- headache

Other symptoms for adults specific to iron deficiency may present, such as alopecia, dry hair or skin, koilonychia, atrophic glossitis, or even restless legs syndrome.[29] They also may present with pica, which is described as the behavior of ingesting soil, clay, ice, or raw ingredients. Iron deficiency may also affect chronic medical conditions including heart failure[30] and ischemic heart disease.[31] If IDA is related to blood loss, one may be hemodynamically unstable which must be addressed acutely.

DIAGNOSIS

The initial step in the workup of IDA is a complete blood count. If the hematocrit is low, the next step is analysis of the MCV. Although IDA is the most common cause of microcytic anemia, up to 40% of patients with normocytic anemia will have a component of iron deficiency. One such diagnostic approach after considering iron deficiency in folks with an MCV less than 95% (which still has a sensitivity of 97.6%) is described in.[32] The most accurate test of diagnosing IDA is ferritin, but caution is advised in inflammatory conditions that may increase ferritin as it is an acute phase reactant. Other tests that can be considered are soluble transferrin receptor and erythrocyte protoporphyrin testing. A bone marrow biopsy is considered the gold standard for IDA.

SEARCH FOR AN UNDERLYING CAUSE

Patients with conditions for bleeding, which have included both genetic inheritable causes, such as von Willebrand disease and also anatomical causes such as gynecological and gastrointestinal causes, should have those worked up and treated. A referral for subspecialist for workup and procedures may be needed. The American Gastroenterological Association in 2020 recommended bidirectional endoscopy in asymptomatic postmenopausal women and men with IDA over no endoscopy.[33] The goal is to look for the source of the bleeding and include the clinical picture (such as gastrointestinal bleeding) as part of the treatment plan.

MANAGEMENT

The goal of treatment of IDA is to replenish iron stores via iron supplementation and to have hemoglobin concentrations return back to normal. Choosing a treatment modality may depend on multiple factors, such as ability to tolerate oral intake, side effects **(Table 2)**.[34,35]

Oral Iron Therapy

There are several forms of oral therapy that can be used to supplement iron, which include ferrous sulfate, ferrous gluconate, and ferrous fumarate. The target dosage of elemental iron to treat IDA is approximately 120 mg of elemental iron per day.[32] For example, 325 mg of ferrous sulfate contains about 105 mg of elemental iron.[36] Optimal dosing of iron can be given on alternate days along with intermediate doses, as compared with prior recommendations.[28] Absorption can be increased by taking iron with ascorbic acid, but this also may lead to increased side gastrointestinal side effects.[37] Side effects may be reduced when iron supplementation is supported by a meal, but this may also result in decreased absorption.[36,38] Studies are still needed to assess if alternate day dosing is more effective. Side effects such as abdominal discomfort, nausea/vomiting, diarrhea, and constipation may affect the patient's adherence to oral iron therapy.

Parenteral Iron Therapy

Intravenous iron therapy can be considered in those patients who cannot tolerate or absorb oral preparations. Examples of patients that may have decreased absorption of iron include those with malabsorption, inflammatory bowel disease, chronic kidney disease, or ongoing blood loss.[39] Main forms of intravenous iron include iron sucrose, ferric gluconate, ferric carboxymaltose, iron isomaltoside-1000, ferumoxytol, and iron dextran. A systemic review in 2016 showed that parenteral iron therapy produced a significantly greater increase in hemoglobin compared with oral iron therapies.[40] However, safety and side effects associated with parenteral iron supplementation have

Table 2
Summaries of iron supplementation treatments and side effects of iron supplementation categories

Treatment	Side Effects
Oral Ferrous Salts	
Ferrous sulfate Ferrous fumarate Ferrous gluconate Iron polymaltose Elemental iron	• Adverse gastrointestinal effects (constipation, nausea, diarrhea) • Decreased absorption with medications/conditions that result in gastric hyposecretion (eg, proton-pump inhibitors, gastrectomy)
Parenteral Iron Administration	
Low molecular weight iron dextran Iron polymaltose Iron sucrose Iron dextran Ferric carboxymaltose Ferric derisomaltose Ferumoxytol Sodium ferric gluconate	• Gastrointestinal side effects (nausea, vomiting) • Infusion reactions (hypersensitivity, urticaria, headache, arthralgias) that require monitoring • Increased risk of infection[34] • Increased risk of anaphylaxis • Restricted to 2nd and 3rd trimester in pregnancy • Skin staining (rare) • Hyperphosphatemia (ferric carboxymaltose)[35]

been a long-standing concern. Iron dextran has been associated with a higher frequency of anaphylactic reactions and multiple recorded fatalities between 1976 and 1996.[41] A systemic review showed that parenteral iron administrations were not associated with serious adverse events, but milder reactions such as urticaria, headache, and arthralgias were not uncommon.[42]

Surveillance and Follow-Up

When treating IDA, there are no standard recommendations for follow-up. One recommendation is to monitor blood counts monthly to see if there is a proper response and increase in hemoglobin.[32] The British Society of Gastroenterology recommends monthly measurements of hemoglobin and iron status for 3 months, then afterwards every 3 months for a year. If symptoms do persist afterward, then further blood tests can be repeated every 3 months.[25] If anemia continues and is unresponsive to iron therapy, further workup to look at other causes of anemia should be considered at this time.

SUMMARY

Primary care physicians are responsible for following preventative screenings for their patients one of which is for colon cancer. Patients may present with related IDA, which must be evaluated as well. Newer screening techniques have provided advancement in the field and with the knowledge of these modalities on how to screen for CRC and treat iron deficiency; the physician will be able to manage these conditions by counseling their patients about the appropriate treatments and resources.

CLINICS CARE POINTS

- The recommended starting age for colon cancer screening now is 45 years of age, but the recommendation is for those with first-degree relatives with colorectal cancer history to still start at age 40 or 10 years before the youngest diagnosed family member.

- Iron deficiency anemia can still be treated with oral iron, but gastrointestinal side effects can be mitigated while still effectively treating the anemia, with taking oral iron less frequently, such as every other day.

DISCLOSURE

The authors have nothing to disclose.

REFERENCES

1. Centers for Disease Control and Prevention. Incidence and relative survival by stage at diagnosis for common cancers. USCS data brief, no. 25. Atlanta, GA: Centers for Disease Control and Prevention, US Department of Health and Human Services; 2021.
2. Centers for Disease Control and Prevention. U.S. Cancer Statistics Colorectal Cancer Stat Bite. US Department of Health and Human Services; 2022. https://www.cdc.gov/cancer/uscs/pdf/USCS-Stat-Bite-Colorectal-508.pdf.
3. Calderwood AH, Lasser KE, Roy HK. Colon adenoma features and their impact on risk of future advanced adenomas and colorectal cancer. World J Gastrointest Oncol 2016;8(12):826–34.

4. Available at: https://www.cdc.gov/cancer/colorectal/statistics/use-screening-tests-BRFSS.htm. Accessed November 1, 2022.
5. Siegel RL, Torre LA, Soerjomataram I, et al. Global patterns and trends in colorectal cancer incidence in young adults. Gut 2019;68:2179–85.
6. Crockett SD, Nagtegaal I. Terminology, molecular features, epidemiology, and management of serrated colorectal neoplasia. Gastroenterology 2019;157: 949–66.e4.
7. United States Preventive Services Task Force. Screening for colorectal cancer: US preventive services task force recommendation statement. JAMA 2021; 325(19):1965–77.
8. Shaukat A, Kahi CJ, Burke CA, et al. ACG clinical guidelines: colorectal cancer screening 2021. Am J Gastroenterol 2021;116:458–79.
9. Wolf A, Fontham ETH, Church TR, et al. Colorectal cancer screening for average-risk adults: 2018 guideline update from the American cancer society. Cancer 2018;68(4):250–81.
10. Segnan N, Armaroli P, Bonelli L, et al. Once-only sigmoidoscopy in colorectal cancer screening: follow-up findings of the Italian randomized control trial – SCORE. J Natl Cancer Inst 2011;17(7):1310–22.
11. Atkin W, Wooldrage K, Parkin DM, et al. Long term effects of once-only flexible sigmoidoscopy screening after 17 years of follow-up: the UK flexible sigmoidoscopy screening randomised controlled trial. Lancet 2017;319:1299–311.
12. Holme Ø, Løberg M, Kalager M, et al, NORCCAP Study Group. Long-term effectiveness of sigmoidoscopy screening on colorectal cancer incidence and mortality in women and men: a randomized trial. Ann Intern Med 2018;168(11):775–82.
13. Kaminski MF, Bretthauer M, Zauber AG, et al. The NordICC Study: rationale and design of a randomized control trial on colonoscopy screening for colorectal cancer. Endoscopy 2012;44(7):695–702.
14. Schoen RE, Pinsky PF, Weissfeld JL, et al. Colorectal-cancer incidence and mortality with screening flexible sigmoidoscopy. N Engl J Med 2012;366(25):2345–57.
15. de Haan MC, van Gelder RE, Graser A, et al. Diagnostic value of CT-colonography as compared to colonoscopy in an asymptomatic screening population: a meta-analysis. Eur Radiol 2011;21(8):1747–63.
16. Konrad G, Katz A. Are medication restrictions before FOBT necessary?: practical advice based on a systematic review of the literature. Can Fam Physician 2012; 58(9):939–48.
17. Lin JS, Perdue LA, Henrikson NB, et al. Screening for colorectal cancer: updated evidence report and systematic review for the US preventive services task force. JAMA 2021;325(19):1978–98.
18. Chiu HM, Chen SL, Yen AM, et al. Effectiveness of fecal immunochemical testing in reducing colorectal cancer mortality from the One Million Taiwanese Screening Program. Cancer 2015;121(18):3221–9.
19. Imperiale TF, Ransohoff DF, Itzkowitz SH, et al. Multitarget stool DNA testing for colorectal-cancer screening. N Engl J Med 2014;370(14):1287–97.
20. Ahlquist DA. Multi-target stool DNA test: a new high bar for noninvasive screening. Dig Dis Sci 2015;60(3):623–33.
21. Song L, Jia J, Xiumei P, et al. The performance of the SEPT9 gene methylation assay and a comparison with other CRC screening tests: A meta-analysis. Sci Rep 2017;7(1):3032.
22. U.S. Food & Drug Administration Post -Approval Studies Database. https://www.accessdata.fda.gov/scripts/cdrh/cfdocs/cfpma/pma_pas.cfm?t_id=505162&c_id=3927. Accessed November 7, 2022.

23. Tool, based on 2021 submission data (1999-2019): U.S. Department of Health and Human Services, Centers for Disease Control and Prevention and National Cancer Institute. Available at: https://www.cdc.gov/cancer/dataviz, Accessed November 1, 2022.

24. Stevens GA, Paciorek CJ, Flores-Urrutia MC, et al. National, regional, and global estimates of anaemia by severity in women and children for 2000-19: a pooled analysis of population-representative data. Lancet Global Health 2022;10:e627–39.

25. Snook J, Bhala N, Beales I, et al. British Society of Gastroenterology guidelines for the management of iron deficiency anaemia in adults. Gut 2021;70(11):2030–51.

26. Cappelini MD, Musallam KM, Taher AT. Iron deficiency anaemia revisited. J Intern Med 2020;287(2):153–70.

27. Kumar A, Sharma E, Marley A, et al. Iron deficiency anaemia: pathophysiology, assessment, practical management. BMJ Open Gastroenterol 2022;9(1):e000759.

28. Pasricha S, Tye-Din J, Muckenthaler MU, et al. Iron deficiency. Lancet 2021;397: 233–48.

29. Andrews NC. Disorders of iron metabolism. N Engl J Med 1999;341:1986–95.

30. Grote Beverborg N, van der Wal HH, Klip IT, et al. Differences in clinical profile and outcomes of low iron storage vs defective iron utilization in patients with heart failure: results from the DEFINE-HF and BIOSTAT-CHF studies. JAMA Cardiol 2019;4:696–701.

31. Perera CA, Biggers RP, Robertson A. Deceitful red-flag: angina secondary to iron deficiency anaemia as a presenting complaint for underlying malignancy. BMJ Case Rep 2019;12:e229942.

32. Short MW, Domagalski JW. Iron deficiency anemia: evaluation and treatment. Am Fam Physician 2013;87(2):98–104.

33. Ko CW, Siddique SM, Patel A, et al. AGA clinical practice guidelines on the gastrointestinal evaluation of iron deficiency anemia. Gastroenterology 2020; 149(3):1085–94.

34. Shah AA, Donovan K, Seeley C, et al. Risk of infection associated with administration of intravenous iron: a systematic review and meta-analysis. JAMA Netw Open 2021;4(11):e2133935.

35. Glaspy JA, Lim-Watson MZ, Libre MA, et al. Hypophosphatemia associated with intravenous iron therapies for iron deficiency anemia: a systematic literature review. Therapeut Clin Risk Manag 2020;16:245–9.

36. World Health Organization. Iron deficiency anaemia: assessment, prevention, and control: a guide for programme managers. Geneva, Switzerland: World Health Organization; 2001.

37. Moretti D, Goede JS, Zeder C, et al. Oral iron supplements increase hepcidin and decrease iron absorption from daily or twice-daily doses in iron-depleted young women. Blood 2015;126:1981–9.

38. Sonoda S. Iron deficiency anemia: guidelines from the american gastroenterological association. Am Fam Physician 2021;104(2):211–2.

39. Lopez A, Cacoub P, Macdougall IC, et al. Iron deficiency anemia. Lancet 2016; 382:907–16.

40. Clevenger B, Gurusamy K, Klein AA, et al. Systematic review and meta-analysis of iron therapy in anaemic adults without chronic kidney disease: updated and abridged Cochrane review. Eur J Heart Fail 2016;18:774–85.

41. Faich G, Strobos J. Sodium ferric gluconate complex in sucrose: safer intravenous iron therapy than iron dextrans. Am J Kidney Dis 1999;33:464–70.

42. Avni T, Bieber A, Grossman A, et al. The safety of intravenous iron preparations: systematic review and meta-analysis. Mayo Clin Proc 2015;90:12–23.

Gut Microbiome and Dietar Considerations

John Damianos, MD[a], Parvathi Perumareddi, DO[b,c],*

KEYWORDS

- Gut microbiome • Microbiota • Gut health • Dysbiosis • Probiotic

KEY POINTS

- The gut microbiome consists of a massive collection of microorganisms in the gastrointestinal tract functioning as its own organ system aiding in digestive, metabolic, and immunologic processes.
- The microbiome is affected by genetic and environmental factors beginning from birth throughout the lifespan, with environmental factors such as diet playing a more prominent role.
- Disruption of the microbiome can result in proinflammatory disease states affecting all organ systems and predisposing to chronic diseases.
- Interventions to improve diversity of the microbiome and support a prohealth state include changes in diet and physical activity, reduction of stress, and restriction of certain medications.

INTRODUCTION
The Gut Microbiome

The gut microbiota comprises a vast network of approximately 100 trillion microorganisms—bacteria, viruses, fungi, archaea, and protozoa—that colonize the gastrointestinal tract. These organisms function as a unique organ system, interacting with intestinal luminal antigens and the intestinal mucosa. They interface directly or indirectly with many organ systems including the immune system, endocrine system, and nervous system. The composition of the microbiota varies throughout the course of the gastrointestinal tract (and is affected by many factors including genetics, diet, environment, and medications).[1] Furthermore, the microbiome is dynamic, constantly evolving in structure and function in response to environmental stimuli, with even circadian and diurnal changes.[2]

[a] Division of Gastroenterology and Hepatology, Mayo Clinic, 200 First Street Southwest, Rochester, MN 55905, USA; [b] Department of Medicine, Florida Atlantic University, Boca Raton, FL, USA; [c] Charles E Schmidt College of Medicine- Florida Atlantic University, 777 Glades Road, Boca Raton, FL 33431, USA
* Corresponding author. Charles E Schmidt College of Medicine- Florida Atlantic University, 777 Glades Road, Boca Raton, FL 33431.
E-mail address: pperumar@health.fau.edu

Prim Care Clin Office Pract 50 (2023) 493–505
https://doi.org/10.1016/j.pop.2023.04.001
0095-4543/23/© 2023 Elsevier Inc. All rights reserved.

primarycare.theclinics.com

Functions of the Microbiota

The gut microbiota exerts effects both locally and systemically. It plays an important role in digestion and metabolism, such as fermenting poorly digestible carbohydrates into short-chain fatty acids, regulating lipid and protein metabolism, regulating bile acid metabolism, synthesizing essential vitamins and nutrients (eg, vitamins K and B components), and breaking down polyphenols for systemic absorption. Another crucial role of the microbiota is maintaining homeostasis of the intestinal mucosal milieu. A healthy microbiome provides defense against invasion by pathogenic bacteria due to secretion of mucus, antimicrobial peptides, and immunoglobulins. Similarly, a healthy microbiome maintains a robust gut epithelial barrier, preventing translocation of pathogenic organisms and toxins. The microbiota also plays a critical role in entrainment of the immune system. The microorganisms and their byproducts interface directly with luminal antigens and the mucosa-associated lymphoid tissues to direct immune responses both locally and systemically. Other important systemic effects of the microbiota include production of hormones and neurotransmitters (eg, serotonin) and metabolism of medications.[3]

Eubiosis and Dysbiosis

A healthy microbiome (broadly termed *eubiosis*) contributes to health, whereas a disrupted microbiome (*dysbiosis*) contributes to illness. Defining a normal microbiome is challenging due to the wide variability in composition across geographic location and factors such as diet and the exposome.[4,5] However, several factors have been identified that reflect a healthy microbiome, including diversity, stability and resilience, absence of pathogenic organisms, and absence of bacterial overgrowth. Low diversity of the microbiota has consistently been associated with adverse health outcomes including inflammatory bowel disease (IBD), *Clostridioides difficile* colitis, obesity, and cancers.[6] Stability of the microbiome refers to the ability of the microbiota to maintain itself in the face of physiologic stressors, and resilience is its ability to recover from these stressors.[7] Because the microbiota interface directly with the immune system, the balance of beneficial, antiinflammatory organisms and pathogenic, proinflammatory organisms contribute to immune activation within the intestine and systemically. For example, a high *Firmicutes* to *Bacteroidetes* ratio has been demonstrated in metabolic disorders,[8] whereas abundance of *Akkermansia muciniphila* is protective against obesity.[9] Similarly, overgrowth of pathogenic species creates a proinflammatory intestinal milieu that is associated with many systemic and inflammatory disorders.[10]

Taken together, the dysbiotic microbiome is characterized by an inflammatory milieu that damages the gut mucosal barrier, causing increased intestinal permeability. Increased permeability allows for the translocation of bacterial products and environmental antigens and toxins (termed metabolic endotoxemia). Bacterial components such as lipopolysaccharide are highly immunogenic, inducing a robust inflammatory response. Similarly, antigenic infiltration of the bloodstream can, in genetically susceptible individuals, trigger an immune cascade that can culminate in systemic inflammation and the development of metabolic and immune-mediated diseases.[11,12] Clearly, perturbations in the microbiota lead to disordered microbial-host interactions, which have been associated with a variety of chronic disease states.[13]

Factors that Affect the Gut Microbiota

Establishment and entrainment of the microbiota begin prenatally and continue throughout life, influenced by several host and extrinsic factors. Although much of the composition of the microbiota is related to environmental exposures, there are genetic influences that do contribute.[14] In the prenatal period, maternal obesity, diet, medications, and health status influence the composition of the vaginal microbiota, which provides most of the organisms that colonize the infant on vaginal delivery. Mode of delivery (ie, vaginal or cesarean) provides one of the strongest contributions to early-life intestinal colonization.[15] Infants born by vaginal delivery versus C-section display radically differing microbiota, with vaginally born infants displaying higher levels of vaginal flora such as beneficial *Lactobacilli* and *Bifidobacteria*, whereas C-section–born infants have higher levels of pathogenic organisms such as *Klebsiella* and *Enterococcus*.[16] Owing largely to the critical role of the infant microbiota on immune entrainment, infants born via C-section have higher rates of obesity, allergic diseases, and immune-mediated diseases including type I diabetes and celiac disease.[17,18] Similarly, infant diet (breastfed vs formula-fed) represents another key contributor to early microbiome function. Breastfed infants display higher microbial diversity and greater abundance of beneficial organisms, namely *Bifidobacteria*. Formula-fed infants on the other hand have more pathogenic organisms (such as *C difficile*), bacterial overgrowth, and increased intestinal permeability.[19,20] And similar to mode of delivery, feeding type has lifelong health implications, with formula-fed infants at higher risk of obesity, nonalcoholic fatty liver disease, and other metabolic conditions.[15,20] Past infancy, environment is a major contributor to the composition and function of the microbiota. Broadly, more Westernized cultures have microbiota characterized by reduced diversity, abundance of pathogenic species, loss of beneficial bacteria, and increased intestinal permeability.[15] Immigration to Westernized countries rapidly induces these changes, and these changes are accentuated with each generation.[21] Urbanization (associated with greater hygiene, more antibiotic use, pollution, and processed foods) is associated with a more Western-type microbiome, which has also been associated with the development of chronic noncommunicable diseases.[22,23] Exposures to nature and animals, on the other hand, supports a healthy microbiome and may even protect against Crohn disease.[24] Diet is another one of the major determinants of the microbiota. A Western-style diet characterized by high trans and saturated fat, refined carbohydrates, processed and ultraprocessed foods, and low fiber and omega-3 fatty acids has consistently been associated with a proinflammatory microbiota characterized by reduced diversity and stability, overabundance of pathogenic species, production of toxic metabolites, and loss of gut mucosal barrier integrity. This dietary pattern is associated with the development of chronic noncommunicable diseases.[25,26] Conversely, plant-based diets rich in diverse fibers are consistently associated with favorable health outcomes.[27] Arguably the most significant benefit of plant-based diets derives from short-chain fatty acids (SCFA) derived via the microbiota. Poorly digestible polysaccharides such as fiber and resistant reach the colon, where they are fermented into SCFA, namely acetate, butyrate, and propionate. These SCFA exert myriad local and systemic effects including lowering the luminal pH (thereby protecting against pathogens), strengthening the integrity of the gut mucosal barrier, inhibiting inflammatory responses, modulating enteroendocrine signaling, and exerting epigenetic modifications.[27] Another direct example of diet-microbiome-host interactions comes from the trimethylamine (TMA) pathway. Dietary choline and carnitine (found in red meat, fish, poultry, eggs) favors specific microbiota that metabolize these factors into TMA, which is subsequently taken up in the portal circulation and ultimately the liver, where flavin-dependent monooxygenase isoforms 1 and 3 convert TMA into TMAO. TMAO has been implicated in the development of endothelial injury and atherosclerosis, ultimately leading to myocardial infarction, stroke, and heart failure.[28] Levels of TMAO can be reduced significantly within 1 week of switching to a vegan diet.[29]

Integration of fermented foods into the diet such as yogurt, kimchi, and kombucha has been found to reduce inflammatory markers in healthy individuals[30]; this is thought to be related to an increase in microbial diversity and enrichment of beneficial SCFA-producing species. This reduction in systemic inflammation may reduce the risk of inflammatory conditions such as diabetes and cardiovascular disease (**Fig. 1**).

In addition to diet, several lifestyle factors contribute to the health of the microbiome. Tobacco and alcohol, for example, are detrimental to the microbiota, predisposing to a proinflammatory milieu.[31] Stress and psychiatric disorders are also associated with proinflammatory microbiota.[32] Exercise on the other hand has favorable effects on the microbiota.[33]

Another important modifiable contributor to the microbiota is medications. Nonsteroidal anti-inflammatory drugs (NSAIDs) and proton pump inhibitors, for example, alter microbiome composition, and the latter is associated with an increased risk of enteric infection, including with *C difficile*.[34] The most profound perturbations to the microbiota, however, come from antibiotic use. Antibiotic use in infancy and early childhood increases the risk of obesity, allergic and atopic diseases, and potentially immune-mediated and infectious diseases.[35] Even later in life, antibiotics reduce microbial diversity; impair the gut mucosal barrier; promote antibiotic resistance; and increase the risk of obesity, IBD, irritable bowel syndrome (IBS), *C difficile*, colorectal cancer, nonalcoholic fatty liver disease, immune-mediated diseases, depression, and dementia, among others.[36]

Finally, the microbiota changes with age, and health of the microbiota may affect the course of aging.[37,38]

The Microbiota and Disease States

Dysbiosis has been implicated in a wide range of disease states across organ systems (**Fig. 2**, **Table 1**).[39]

Therapeutic Modulation of the Microbiota

Various lifestyle modifications have consistently proved to favorably alter the microbiota, in turn improving health outcomes.

Diet

The most predictable and reliable way to influence the microbiota is via diet.[26] The following dietary principles promote diversity, stability, and an antiinflammatory milieu:

- Plant-based diets (eg, Mediterranean diet, vegetarian diet, vegan diet)
- Animal fats
- Omega-3 fatty acids
- Fiber
- Fermented foods
- Polyphenols
- Omega-3 fatty acids and plant fats
- Emulsifiers/additives (eg, maltodextrin, titanium dioxide, carrageenans)
- Refined carbohydrates
- Ultraprocessed foods

Lifestyle

Apart from diet, the following are recommended to support a healthy microbiome:

- Avoidance of smoking
- Limit alcohol (particularly spirits)

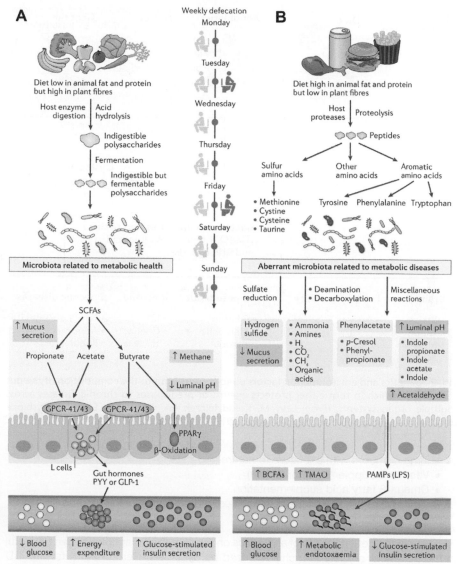

Fig. 1. Healthy and unhealthy dietary patterns affect the microbiota in distinct ways, with healthy, plant-based, high-fiber diets increasing short-chain fatty acids and reducing local and systemic inflammation and unhealthy diets featuring animal products, saturated fats, refined carbohydrates, and ultraprocessed foods contributing to proinflammatory local and systemic milieu by damaging the microbiota and gut epithelial barrier. (*A*) Low Animal Fat and Protein/ High Plant fiber diet. (*B*) High Animal Fat and Protein/Low Plant fiber diet. (*From* Fan Y, Pedersen O. Gut microbiota in human metabolic health and disease. *Nat Rev Microbiol.* 2021;19(1):55-71.)

- Regular aerobic exercise (150 minutes of moderate-to-vigorous activity per week)
- Treatment of stress, anxiety, depression
- Sleep hygiene

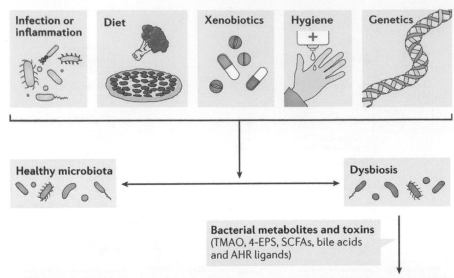

Fig. 2. Genetics and environmental factors directly contribute to the composition of the gut microbiota, which in turn either protects against or predisposes to chronic diseases across multiple organ systems. (*From* Levy M, Kolodziejczyk AA, Thaiss CA, Elinav E. Dysbiosis and the immune system. Nat Rev Immunol. 2017;17(4):219-232.)

- Time outdoors with exposure to nature and pets
- Vitamin D supplementation (if low)
- Omega-3 fatty acid supplementation
- Limit use of broad-spectrum antibiotics, proton pump inhibitors, and NSAIDs

Antibiotics

Because of the potent effects of antibiotics on the microbiota, antibiotics can be useful in the treatment of disorders characterized by dysbiosis. Certain patients with IBD such as Crohn disease with perianal involvement may benefit from treatment with antibiotics.[40] Certain disorders of gut-brain interaction such as IBS and functional dyspepsia respond well to the nonabsorbed antibiotic rifaximin.[41,42] Rifaximin is also used in the treatment of hepatic encephalopathy and small intestinal bacterial overgrowth.[43,44] In addition to its antimicrobial effects, rifaximin may also exert antiinflammatory effects and strengthen the gut mucosal barrier[45] (**Fig. 3**).

Probiotics

Probiotics are defined as "live microorganisms which when administered in adequate amounts confer a health benefit on the host."[46] Interest in and use of probiotics are rapidly expanding; however, due to lack of Food and Drug Administration (FDA) oversight regarding supplements, there are unique challenges and considerations with respect to recommending probiotics. The foremost consideration with respect to

Table 1
Disease states implicated in dysbiosis

Central nervous system	• Parkinson disease
	• Alzheimer disease
	• Multiple sclerosis
	• Anxiety
	• Depression
	• PTSD
Cardiovascular	• Atherosclerotic cardiovascular disease
	• Hypertension
	• Hyperlipidemia
Pulmonary	• Asthma
	• COPD
	• Interstitial lung disease
Rheumatologic	• Systemic lupus erythematosus
	• Rheumatoid arthritis
	• Seronegative spondyloarthropathies
	• Sjögren disease
	• Systemic sclerosis
Endocrine	• Diabetes mellitus
	• Thyroid disorders
Renal	• Chronic kidney disease
Genitourinary	• Bacterial vaginosis
	• Recurrent UTIs
	• Preterm birth
	• Preeclampsia
Oncologic	• Colorectal cancer
	• Liver cancer
	• Breast cancer
	• Prostate cancer
Skin	• Psoriasis
	• Atopic dermatitis
	• Acne vulgaris
Hepatic	• Nonalcoholic fatty liver disease
	• Cirrhosis
	• Autoimmune hepatitis
	• Primary biliary cholangitis
	• Primary sclerosing cholangitis
Gastrointestinal	• Inflammatory bowel disease
	• Irritable bowel syndrome
	• Small intestinal bacterial overgrowth
	• Celiac disease

Abbreviations: COPD, chronic obstructive pulmonary disease; PTSD, posttraumatic stress disorder; UTIs, urinary tract infections.

probiotics is strain specificity. Although some properties of probiotics may be species or even genus specific, it is clear that even within a species, strains exert different biologic activity. An example of a probiotic bacterium is *Bifidobacterium longum* 35624 (denoting *genus*, *species*, and *strain*). Other considerations include colony forming units (CFU), which partly determine the survivability of the organisms within the gastrointestinal tract. Each strain will require a unique CFU to be effective, although typically 10 to 100 million CFU/g is the minimum requirement to achieve a therapeutic 1 to 10 million CFU/g in the colon.[47] Related, some probiotics contain a single strain, whereas

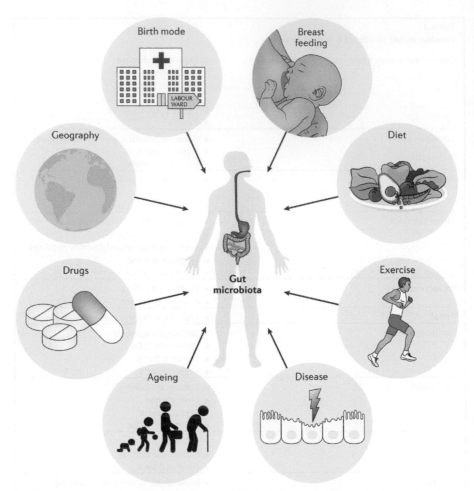

Fig. 3. Numerous environmental factors contribute to the composition and function of the gut microbiota. (*From* Quigley EMM. Gut microbiome as a clinical tool in gastrointestinal disease management: are we there yet?. Nat Rev Gastroenterol Hepatol. 2017;14(5):315-320.)

others have several. Certain strains require refrigeration, whereas others do not. Timing of probiotic administration with relation to meals and composition of the meal may also affect survivability in the gastrointestinal tract.[48] It is also important to note that most probiotics do not colonize the gut but exert their effects locally through interaction with the intestinal luminal environment; this also means that the therapeutic effects typically end after stopping the probiotic.[49]

Perhaps the strongest data for probiotics arise from prevention of antibiotic-associated diarrhea.[50] Other indications include the prevention of travelers diarrhea, treatment of occasional symptoms of diarrhea, constipation, and bloating, prevention of *C difficile*, prevention and treatment of hepatic encephalopathy, treatment of ulcerative colitis and pouchitis, treatment of disorders of gut-brain interaction (eg, IBS, functional dyspepsia, and functional abdominal pain), weight management, dyslipidemia, and anxiety and depression. In counseling patients on probiotic use, they should

Table 2 Supplements	
Prebiotic	"Substrate that is selectively utilized by host microorganisms conferring a health benefit"[46]
Probiotic	"Live microorganisms which when administered in adequate amounts confer a health benefit on the host"[46]
Synbiotic	"A mixture comprising live microorganisms and substrate(s) selectively utilized by host microorganisms that confers a health benefit on the host"[53]
Postbiotic	"Preparation of inanimate microorganisms and/or their components that confers a health benefit on the host"[54]

be directed toward strain studies for the particular indication and sold by a reputable company. Probiotics resources such as the International Scientific Association for Probiotics and Prebiotics and the Alliance for Education on Probiotics are useful in guiding patients and clinicians.[51,52]

Related to probiotics, other related therapies aiming to enrich the microbiota are defined in **Table 2**:

Fecal microbiota transplantation. In fecal microbiota transplantation (FMT), stool from a healthy donor (or donors) is administered (via capsules or endoscopically) to the patient with the goal of alleviating the dysbiosis underlying a particular disease. Currently, the only FDA-sanctioned indication for FMT is for the prevention of recurrent *C difficile* infection (it can also be used for first episodes of *C difficile* infection if fulminant).[55] FMT also has emerging data for ulcerative colitis, IBS, and hepatic encephalopathy and is being investigated for a wide variety of conditions from obesity to autism spectrum disorder.

Newer microbiome-targeted therapies. In addition to the aforementioned interventions, there are newer experimental microbiome-based therapies that aim to provide a more targeted approach to alleviating dysbiosis. These therapies include bacterial components and derivatives, live biotherapeutics, engineered probiotics, and phage therapies. REBYOTA (fecal microbiota, live-jslm) is the first FDA-approved live biotherapeutic, with indication for the treatment of recurrent *C difficile* infection.[56]

It is important to note that a variety of companies offer direct-to-consumer products that claim to sequence the microbiota based on stool samples; this is not recommended at this time (outside of clinical research), for several reasons including that the stool microbiome is different from the luminal microbiome, the microbiota varies in composition across all parts of the gastrointestinal tract, composition of the microbiota also varies dramatically throughout the day and in response to external stimuli, there are no standard references for a normal microbiome, and sequencing techniques differ widely across companies.[57,58]

CLINICS CARE POINTS

- Discuss diet and specific components such as diversity, plant-based diets, omega-3 fatty acids, fermented foods, and fiber to enrich the microbiota and support health.
- Counsel patients to minimize highly processed foods, avoid tobacco, and limit alcohol consumption.

- Emphasize lifestyle modifications including stress reduction, increased physical activity/exercise, and exposure to outdoors and pets.
- Limit use of certain medications such as broad-spectrum antibiotics, proton pump inhibitors, and NSAIDs unless clearly indicated.

DISCLOSURE

The authors have no funding to disclose.

REFERENCES

1. Vuik FER, Dicksved J, Lam SY, et al. Composition of the mucosa-associated microbiota along the entire gastrointestinal tract of human individuals. United Eur Gastroenterol J 2019;7(7):897–907.
2. Takayasu L, Suda W, Takanashi K, et al. Circadian oscillations of microbial and functional composition in the human salivary microbiome. DNA Res 2017;24(3): 261–70.
3. Jandhyala SM. Role of the normal gut microbiota. World J Gastroenterol 2015; 21(29):8787.
4. He Y, Wu W, Zheng H-M, et al. Regional variation limits applications of Healthy Gut Microbiome Reference Ranges and disease models. Nat Med 2018;24(10): 1532–5.
5. Yatsunenko T, Rey FE, Manary MJ, et al. Human gut microbiome viewed across age and geography. Nature 2012;486(7402):222–7.
6. Lozupone CA, Stombaugh JI, Gordon JI, et al. Diversity, stability and resilience of the human gut microbiota. Nature 2012;489(7415):220–30.
7. Bäckhed F, Fraser CM, Ringel Y, et al. Defining a healthy human gut microbiome: Current concepts, future directions, and clinical applications. Cell Host Microbe 2012;12(5):611–22.
8. Carding S, Verbeke K, Vipond DT, et al. Dysbiosis of the gut microbiota in disease. Microb Ecol Health Dis 2015;26. https://doi.org/10.3402/mehd.v26.26191.
9. Ottman N, Geerlings SY, Aalvink S, et al. Action and function of Akkermansia Muciniphila in microbiome ecology, Health and Disease. Best Pract Res Clin Gastroenterol 2017;31(6):637–42.
10. Rizos E, Pyleris E, Pimentel M, et al. Small intestine bacterial overgrowth can form an indigenous proinflammatory environment in the duodenum: A prospective study. Microorganisms 2022;10(5):960.
11. Arrieta MC. Alterations in intestinal permeability. Gut 2006;55(10):1512–20.
12. Teshima CW, Meddings JB. The measurement and clinical significance of intestinal permeability. Curr Gastroenterol Rep 2008;10(5):443–9.
13. Bäckhed F, Fraser CM, Ringel Y, et al. Defining a healthy human gut microbiome: Current concepts, future directions, and clinical applications. Cell Host Microbe 2012;12(5):611–22.
14. Goodrich JK, Waters JL, Poole AC, et al. Human genetics shape the gut microbiome. Cell 2014;159(4):789–99.
15. Jian C, Carpén N, Helve O, et al. Early-life gut microbiota and its connection to metabolic health in children: Perspective on ecological drivers and need for quantitative approach. EBioMedicine 2021;69:103475.

16. Reyman M, van Houten MA, van Baarle D, et al. Impact of delivery mode-associated gut microbiota dynamics on health in the first year of life. Nat Commun 2019;10(1). https://doi.org/10.1038/s41467-019-13014-7.

17. Isolauri E. Development of healthy gut microbiota early in life. J Paediatr Child Health 2012;48:1–6.

18. Francino MP. Birth mode-related differences in gut microbiota colonization and immune system development. Ann Nutr Metabol 2018;73(Suppl. 3):12–6.

19. Azad MB, Konya T, Maughan H, et al. Gut Microbiota of Healthy Canadian infants: Profiles by mode of delivery and infant diet at 4 months. Can Med Assoc J 2013; 185(5):385–94.

20. O'Sullivan A, Farver M, Smilowitz JT. Article commentary: The influence of early infant-feeding practices on the intestinal microbiome and body composition in infants. Nutr Metab Insights 2015;8s1. https://doi.org/10.4137/nmi.s29530.

21. Vangay P, Johnson AJ, Ward TL, et al. US immigration westernizes the human gut microbiome. Cell 2018;175(4). https://doi.org/10.1016/j.cell.2018.10.029.

22. Zuo T, Kamm MA, Colombel J-F, et al. Urbanization and the gut microbiota in health and inflammatory bowel disease. Nat Rev Gastroenterol Hepatol 2018; 15(7):440–52.

23. Li X, Stokholm J, Brejnrod A, et al. The infant gut resistome associates with E. coli, environmental exposures, gut microbiome maturity, and asthma-associated bacterial composition. Cell Host Microbe 2021;29(6). https://doi.org/10.1016/j.chom.2021.03.017.

24. Tun HM, Konya T, Takaro TK, et al. Exposure to household furry pets influences the gut microbiota of infants at 3–4 months following various birth scenarios. Microbiome 2017;5(1). https://doi.org/10.1186/s40168-017-0254-x.

25. David LA, Maurice CF, Carmody RN, et al. Diet rapidly and reproducibly alters the human gut microbiome. Nature 2013;505(7484):559–63.

26. Fan Y, Pedersen O. Gut Microbiota in human metabolic health and disease. Nat Rev Microbiol 2020;19(1):55–71.

27. Rooks MG, Garrett WS. Gut microbiota, metabolites and host immunity. Nat Rev Immunol 2016;16(6):341–52.

28. Tilg H. A gut feeling about thrombosis. N Engl J Med 2016;374(25):2494–6.

29. Argyridou S, Davies MJ, Biddle GJ, et al. Evaluation of an 8-week vegan diet on plasma trimethylamine-N-oxide and postchallenge glucose in adults with dysglycemia or obesity. J Nutr 2021;151(7):1844–53.

30. Wastyk HC, Fragiadakis GK, Perelman D, et al. Gut-microbiota-targeted diets modulate human immune status. Cell 2021;184(16):4137–53.

31. Capurso G, Lahner E. The interaction between smoking, alcohol and the gut microbiome. Best Pract Res Clin Gastroenterol 2017;31(5):579–88.

32. Kelly JR, Kennedy PJ, Cryan JF, et al. Breaking down the barriers: The gut microbiome, intestinal permeability and stress-related psychiatric disorders. Front Cell Neurosci 2015;9. https://doi.org/10.3389/fncel.2015.00392.

33. Sohail MU, Yassine HM, Sohail A, et al. Impact of physical exercise on gut microbiome, inflammation, and the pathobiology of metabolic disorders. Rev Diabet Stud 2019;15(1):35–48.

34. Le Bastard Q, Al-Ghalith GA, Grégoire M, et al. Systematic review: Human gut dysbiosis induced by non-antibiotic prescription medications. Aliment Pharmacol Ther 2017;47(3):332–45.

35. Vangay P, Ward T, Gerber JS, et al. Antibiotics, pediatric dysbiosis, and disease. Cell Host Microbe 2015;17(5):553–64.

36. Ramirez J, Guarner F, Bustos Fernandez L, et al. Antibiotics as major disruptors of gut microbiota. Front Cell Infect Microbiol 2020;10. https://doi.org/10.3389/fcimb. 2020.572912.

37. Leite G, Pimentel M, Barlow GM, et al. Age and the aging process significantly alter the small bowel microbiome. Cell Rep 2021;36(13):109765.

38. Zapata HJ, Quagliarello VJ. The microbiota and microbiome in aging: Potential implications in health and age-related diseases. J Am Geriatr Soc 2015;63(4): 776–81.

39. Levy M, Kolodziejczyk AA, Thaiss CA, et al. Dysbiosis and the immune system. Nat Rev Immunol 2017;(4):219–32.

40. Ledder O, Turner D. Antibiotics in IBD: Still a role in the biological era? Inflamm Bowel Dis 2018;24(8):1676–88.

41. Rifaximin for irritable bowel syndrome without constipation. N Engl J Med 2011; 364(15):1467–8.

42. Shah A, Gurusamy SR, Hansen T, et al. Concomitant irritable bowel syndrome does not influence the response to antimicrobial therapy in patients with functional dyspepsia. Dig Dis Sci 2021;67(6):2299–309.

43. Blaney H, DeMorrow S. Hepatic encephalopathy: Thinking beyond ammonia. Clinical Liver Disease 2022;19(1):21–4.

44. Wang J, Zhang L, Hou X. Efficacy of rifaximin in treating with small intestine bacterial overgrowth: A systematic review and meta-analysis. Expet Rev Gastroenterol Hepatol 2021;15(12):1385–99.

45. Patel VC, Lee S, McPhail MJW, et al. Rifaximin-α reduces gut-derived inflammation and mucin degradation in cirrhosis and encephalopathy: RIFSYS randomised controlled trial. J Hepatol 2022;76(2):332–42.

46. Hill C, Guarner F, Reid G, et al. The International Scientific Association for Probiotics and prebiotics consensus statement on the scope and appropriate use of the term probiotic. Nat Rev Gastroenterol Hepatol 2014;11(8):506–14.

47. Naissinger da Silva M, Tagliapietra BL, Flores Vdo, et al. In vitro test to evaluate survival in the gastrointestinal tract of commercial probiotics. Curr Res Food Sci 2021;4:320–5.

48. Tompkins T, Mainville I, Arcand Y. The impact of meals on a probiotic during transit through a model of the human upper gastrointestinal tract. Benef Microbes 2011;2(4):295–303.

49. Bezkorovainy A. Probiotics: Determinants of survival and growth in the gut. Am J Clin Nutr 2001;73(2). https://doi.org/10.1093/ajcn/73.2.399s.

50. Liao W, Chen C, Wen T, et al. Probiotics for the prevention of antibiotic-associated diarrhea in adults. J Clin Gastroenterol 2020;55(6):469–80.

51. Kc. ISAPP - International Scientific Association for Probiotics and prebiotics. International Scientific Association for Probiotics and Prebiotics (ISAPP). Available at: https://isappscience.org/. Published January 11, 2023. Accessed February 10, 2023.

52. Alliance for Education on Probiotics . AEProbio. Available at: https://aeprobio. com/. Accessed February 10, 2023.

53. Swanson KS, Gibson GR, Hutkins R, et al. The International Scientific Association for Probiotics and prebiotics (ISAPP) consensus statement on the definition and scope of synbiotics. Nat Rev Gastroenterol Hepatol 2020;17(11):687–701.

54. Salminen S, Collado MC, Endo A, et al. The International Scientific Association of Probiotics and prebiotics (ISAPP) consensus statement on the definition and scope of postbiotics. Nat Rev Gastroenterol Hepatol 2021;18(9):649–67.

55. Kelly CR, Fischer M, Allegretti JR, et al. ACG clinical guidelines: Prevention, diagnosis, and treatment of clostridioides difficile infections. Am J Gastroenterol 2021; 116(6):1124–47.

56. Feuerstadt P, Louie TJ, Lashner B, et al. Ser-109, an oral microbiome therapy for recurrent *clostridioides difficile* infection. N Engl J Med 2022;386(3):220–9.

57. Allaband C, McDonald D, Vázquez-Baeza Y, et al. Microbiome 101: Studying, analyzing, and interpreting gut microbiome data for clinicians. Clin Gastroenterol Hepatol 2019;17(2):218–30.

58. Crits-Christoph A, Suez J. Gut bacteria go on record. Nat Rev Gastroenterol Hepatol 2022;19(9):557–8.

Moving?

Make sure your subscription moves with you!

To notify us of your new address, find your **Clinics Account Number** (located on your mailing label above your name), and contact customer service at:

Email: journalscustomerservice-usa@elsevier.com

800-654-2452 (subscribers in the U.S. & Canada)
314-447-8871 (subscribers outside of the U.S. & Canada)

Fax number: 314-447-8029

Elsevier Health Sciences Division
Subscription Customer Service
3251 Riverport Lane
Maryland Heights, MO 63043

*To ensure uninterrupted delivery of your subscription, please notify us at least 4 weeks in advance of move.

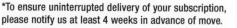

Moving?

Printed and bound by CPI Group (UK) Ltd, Croydon, CR0 4YY

03/10/2024

01040468-0018